THE
BEVERLY
HILLS
DIET

THE BEVERLY HILLS HILLS DIET

BY JUDY MAZEL

WITH SUSAN SHULTZ

MACMILLAN PUBLISHING CO., INC.

NEW YORK

MACMILLAN PUBLISHING CO., INC.
866 THIRD AVENUE, NEW YORK, N.Y. 10022
COLLIER MACMILLAN CANADA, LTD.

Library of Congress Cataloging in Publication Data
Mazel, Judy.
The Beverly Hills diet.
Includes index.
1. Reducing diets. 2. Nutrition. 3. Vegetarianism.
I. Shultz, Susan. II. Title.
RM222.2.M42   613.2'5   81-1520
ISBN 0-02-582600-X   AACR2

10 9 8 7 6

DESIGNED BY JACK MESEROLE

PRINTED IN THE UNITED STATES OF AMERICA

This book is not intended as a substitute
for the medical advice of physicians.
The reader should regularly consult a physician
in matters relating to his or her health and
particularly in respect to any symptoms
that may require diagnosis.

RECIPE CONSULTANT:
JEAN BRADY,
JEAN BRADY COOKING SCHOOL,
SANTA MONICA, CALIFORNIA

Contents

CONTENTS

A Word from the Doctor

It is with great pleasure that I recommend the Beverly Hills Diet to you.

After consulting Judy Mazel for guidance in the art of losing weight, I dropped forty pounds on the healthiest and most enjoyable, *yes enjoyable*, diet I have ever encountered. Perhaps most important, I have kept this weight off through the frantic Beverly Hills holiday season and despite a richly filled summer in the south of France.

Most happily, my health too has prospered. My blood pressure is down and I've thrown away the medicine I used to take to control it. My cholesterol and uric acid levels have dropped and my ulcer has left me in peace.

I have recommended Judy's Beverly Hills Diet to many of my patients, who have thrived on her program just as I have.

It is apparent to me that Judy's "Conscious Combining" represents an important breakthrough approach to weight reduction. This is a program with enormous significance for every person with weight to lose.

The advantages of the Beverly Hills Diet are many. Beverly Hills Dieters are not hungry even in the most concentrated early phases of the diet; thus, the program is easier to adhere to than other so-called quick-weight-loss diets. A nutritional balance is maintained throughout; therefore no artificial supplements are required. The foods provide a high percentage of essential vitamins and minerals, and the mix of fats, carbohydrates, and proteins meets our bodies' needs far better than the traditional "balanced"

American diet. Because the intake of sugar and sodium is minimized, the health of the "Combiner" almost inevitably improves in terms of cholesterol and blood pressure levels, and since fruit is a major component of the program, high energy is an immediate and seemingly lasting by-product as long as "Conscious Combining" is adhered to.

Judy Mazel addresses both the physical and emotional needs of the overweight person. She focuses not only the *effects* of overeating but the *causes* as well, and in the process teaches Beverly Hills Dieters how to use food to their advantage. By reordering the overweight person's approach to eating—introducing Mono Meals and other dietary innovations—she makes us aware of eating as a mental as well as a physical experience and shows us how to control our response to food. Medically, the Beverly Hills Diet seems sound, based as it is on substantial research into the sciences of physiology and enzymology. Certainly, it compares favorably to the lopsided fad diets that have saturated the market in recent years, the one-shot, all-or-nothing measures that have consistently failed to address the long-range needs of dieters.

As I mentioned, I myself have been on the Beverly Hills Diet as have many of my patients. We are all delighted with the results. As a physician I enthusiastically recommend Judy's program to you. It is a sound, effective, and healthy approach to weight loss with results that are unmatched in my experience.

Of course, anyone considering this or any weight reduction program should do so only with the advice and consent of their own physician. And anyone with a chronic ailment should undertake this or any diet only under the direct supervision of their own physician.

VICTOR BENATAR, M.D.
Beverly Hills, California

Acknowledgments

THANK GOD FOR

Susan Shultz for being able to hear it

Margie Platt, Herman Platt, and Oscar Janiger for their big shoulders

The Beverly Hills Hotel for providing refuge from my frantic world

Harry Langdon for giving me another chance

Galanos for supplying the best props a girl ever had

Gary Rome for a gorgeous red dress

Cindy Griffith, who kept smiling no matter how many papers she had to pick up

The Kahala Hilton for providing inspiration

The staff of the Kahala Hilton for keeping us well fed and happy

Toni Lopopolo, my editor, for recognizing the power of the hip-bone and proving it

Charles Kivowitz for blessing the pineapple

Marlena Brauer for infinite wisdom

Norman Brokaw and Irene Webb, for spotting a good thing

Lynn Myers for catching me in the act and helping put together the pieces

Carol Green for undying enthusiasm

Jane Weiss, Joan Jones, and Linda Benvin for tireless fingers

The Regency Hotel, my home away from home, and Mr. Fernandez

Excel Limo for never blinking an eye, no matter what the request

Melinda Rosenthal for arriving on the scene and letting there be peace

Merryl Rosenthal for achieving her goal of a gorgeous body in record time

Donna Smith and Linda McCrea and their coffee, tea, and sleep

Bobbi Cowan for making me realize I could do it

Edna Robinson for becoming a vegetarian

Scott Gershen and the role he played in making nutrition a part of my life

Herbert Shelton for having written his book

Sondra Karl for her get-well present

My mother for caring I was fat

The Chicago diet doctor who gave me my first diet pill

And each and everyone of you who entrusted me with your fat and became my "best examples"

Introduction:
Judy Mazel's
Beverly
Hills
Diet

Welcome to the diet phenomenon of the '80s—the diet that first exploded into reality in the heart of Beverly Hills among the movie stars, the jet-setters, and the ultra body conscious who are hardened to flimsy fads. The diet embraced by everyone from "Dallas" star Linda Gray, actress Sally Kellerman, and singer Englebert Humperdinck to hundreds of skinnies shouting the praises of the Beverly Hills Diet—a way of eating that has turned slimhood into a reality. A way of eating I call Conscious Combining.

Entrepreneur Irwin Molasky, of Las Vegas, is spied at a five-hundred-dollar-a-plate benefit dinner spearing watermelon. A film and stage actress is munching popcorn on the way to the set. A La Jolla housewife is popping grapes at her bridge luncheon. A Phoenix business executive is making a meal of baked potatoes at Durant's Steak House, and a New York book editor is packing papayas in her briefcase. What is going on? These people say they're on a diet and they love it. They say they've never felt or looked better . . . and they claim they aren't hungry! Why? They are Conscious Food Combiners. They have discovered Judy Mazel's Beverly Hills Diet.

They are learning about the enzymatic capabilities of their bodies and how this relates to the food they eat. They are learning how to eat what they really like, not what they think they should like. They are discovering a way of eating that has become a way of life.

The Beverly Hills Diet is an exciting adventure into the world of food—a world of tastes, textures, aromas, feelings, and above all, awareness. "Combiners" not only acknowledge their food fantasies, they fulfill them—while they are losing weight. And, for the first time in their lives, they learn how to control *how they feel* by what they eat.

You too can become a Conscious Combiner. You too can learn to eat what you like, what you crave, what you want—without getting fat. You too can learn that getting thin and eating right can be fun.

Diet does not have to mean deprivation. It's no longer necessary to exist on grapefruit, celery sticks, and four-ounce servings of dry fish or skinless chicken. No more light-headedness and sapped energy. No more diet misery. On the Beverly Hills Diet you will lose weight by feeding your body, not by starving it.

On my program there is no calorie counting and no food weighing. Those dreaded nevers mandated by other diets are banished forever. On what other diet can you eat popcorn, pizza, spareribs, cheesecake, and ice cream and still lose weight?

There are no pills, shots, supplements, or additives. Snacking is encouraged. In fact, eating is encouraged. Hunger is abolished.

You will never go hungry on my diet. You can be as compulsive as you need to be. You can eat as much as you want. You can really get full. There are no portion controls. You can eat whenever you want. There are no specific mealtimes. You are not confined to breakfast, lunch, and dinner. You can eat anywhere, anytime: in your car, in your office, while you're talking on the telephone, even while you're standing at the refrigerator door.

This is a diet in its truest Latin definition—meaning a way of life. One that you adapt to your way of life.

The Beverly Hills Diet is an intellectual approach to eating based on physical facts. Food will take on a new meaning. Nothing and everything is fattening. Low-fat milk in your coffee can be far more devastating than a hamburger with everything on it. You will learn that it's not *what* you eat or *how much* you eat but *when* you eat and what you eat together that counts.

The Beverly Hills Diet is an eater's dream come true. You eat anything and everything you want in a safe, controlled environment. You learn how to make even the most so-called fattening foods not fattening. The Beverly Hills Diet teaches you how to make food work for you, not against you. You will begin to embrace food instead of fighting it.

I have devoted my life to making people thin through Conscious Combining and the Beverly Hills Diet, to becoming the skinny voice of America, the diet conscience of the world. The diet did not develop haphazardly. It is the product of a conscious, consuming, intensive effort which spanned years of study, experimentation, and observation. I have reviewed and synthesized the work of scores of scientists, nutritionists, and doctors and applied it first to myself and then to literally hundreds of others—refining, perfecting, simplifying. The result is a program so logical and simple, so forever, you'll wonder why it's just been developed.

The Beverly Hills Diet does not represent an isolated space in time when we're either "on a diet" or "off a diet," a mentality that equates losing weight with suffering.

The Beverly Hills Diet is not a panacea. It does not guarantee that you'll lose a certain number of pounds in a certain number of days. It is not a temporary plan you can adhere to for only a limited amount of time, a rigid regimen that insists on harsh, unbending conformity, that prescribes for all humanity as if it were a single eater. This is a diet for each individual. This is a diet that you make your own.

Food is more than for just right now. More than a taste in the mouth. As you reject the diet regimens of the '60s and the '70s and embrace the Beverly Hills Diet, you let food assume its natural place in your life. By understanding what it is and what it isn't you will learn how to use food rather than abuse it. You will, for the first time in your life, gain control. Total control. For the first time in your life you will give yourself permission—permission to eat, to feel, to enjoy—and in the process, you will lose weight.

The Beverly Hills Diet acknowledges your emotions and how they affect your weight. Food will always be an emotional stopgap, an expression of love, an instant and temporary cure for boredom, sadness, depression, excitement. For those of us to whom food is important, it is really important; it is a critical and integral part of our lives.

We love to eat, we live to eat—but we hate being fat. Being fat is going to bed feeling bad about ourselves and waking up feeling bad about ourselves. It's the last thing on our mind at night and the first thing we think of when we wake up. And it's miserable. As one of my clients points out, although many fatties joke about their size, "Just as for anyone who's suffered, it's not funny."

There exists in all of us, inside every eater, a constant struggle between the skinny self and the fat self—a mind/body split. (See page 52.) We can only resolve this conflict through experience and understanding, acknowledging the excuses we make to rationalize our eating.

Food is memories—happiness, warmth, reward. It's mother—it's love and it's comfort. Try as we might, we just can't give it up. Some of us are almost there—ten, maybe even five pounds away. Yet something always seems to stop us. We punish ourselves; we abuse ourselves; we try one assault after another. We hook onto every new diet promise. We reach out again and again. We lose, we gain. We're up, we're down . . . we blew it. We have three sizes of clothing, and we wake up every morning wondering what diet to start today.

We don't *want* to be fat. But we don't want to give up eating (and all it represents) either.

What so many of us fail to realize, or at least acknowledge, from this miserable treadmill we are on is that we just plain love to eat. And nothing—not behavior modification, not aversion therapy, not even hypnosis—is ever going to change that. This feeling toward food, this love, and this need are as inherent in our personality as any other characteristics. And just as you wouldn't cut off Michelangelo's hands, you can't shut the mouth of an eater either. Haven't you, haven't I, haven't we proved it again and again?

Diets are not realistic. They never become a way of life because rarely, if ever, do they include what we really *want*: the food that made us fat to begin with.

To the seasoned dieter, the mere word "diet" evokes memories of hunger and deprivation, and none of us is going to make deprivation a permanent way of life. Dieting has always been considered a temporary phase, that stopgap before the big bonanza. When it's all over and we can eat anything we want. The grand illusion.

Thus the fat cycle perpetuates itself and life and fat go on. Deprivation or overindulgence. Feast or famine. So, you've blown it; you might as well really blow it. What difference does it make? And so every meal becomes the last supper because tomorrow you are really going to start that new diet, and since that new diet means forever giving up everything you love—all those "last supper" foods—you'd better get them all in today. Because once you start this new "diet" you are never going to blow it again. But tomorrow comes, and it is just like the tomorrow of yesterday, filled with unfulfilled good intentions. No wonder you're not thin. But you keep eating—and feeling guilty. Well, what right do you have to enjoy it? You're fat and getting fatter.

On one thing we can all agree. The old diet prescriptions are, in reality, prescriptions for failure. They simply don't work.

If they did, would twenty-two million women wear a size sixteen or over? Would fat afflict more than seventy million Americans? Would obesity play a role in the deaths of fifty thousand people every year? All this, in spite of our newfound addiction to health, fitness, and feeling good? When what we desperately want to be is thin? Being fat is an obscenity—we are shunted, scorned, and ridiculed. A *failure* for all to see—and mock. Yet we continue to try, and we continue to fail.

This time you are not going to fail because I am not going to take away the one thing that means more to you than being thin—food. I am not going to make you give up *anything* forever; anything, that is, except that excess weight, the guilt that goes along with it, and a few worn-out beliefs about fattening foods and diets. All those foods you love to eat and live to eat will be a part of your life always. You will never have to cheat to have them. You will *never* have to cheat again!

You will give yourself permission to enjoy food, to relish eating. Food will be a top priority in your life, as it should be, without shame, without apology. But instead of food controlling you, you will control it.

Without a plan, we are hopeless, doomed to that seemingly endless cycle of thin/fat, up/down. We need a support system that is active and alive, one that means forever; that enables us to forever blot out the all-consuming diet consciousness that keeps us fat.

Well, tomorrow is here and it is here for you to enjoy because this is what I offer you. A support system that I am going to help you develop. A support system that is unique because it exists within you. A support system you can depend on. A support system that is forever.

Ultimately, the Beverly Hills Diet will become second nature to you—as easy and natural as brushing your teeth. Conscious Combining will be internalized and become Unconscious Combining.

You too can become a Conscious Combiner. You too can share in the brotherhood and sisterhood of skinnies. With this method of eating, you will get thin, and you will stay thin. You will wear the little golden pineapple, my symbol of eternal slimhood, given to my graduates when they reach and maintain their goal.

You will never have to be fat again.

I do not purport to be a medical doctor.
My findings are based on my personal experience
together with those of the hundreds of
successful skinnies who have followed
the tenets of Conscious Combining and
the Beverly Hills Diet.

Granted, my ideas are revolutionary,
but isn't it about time we found a cure for fat?
If medical experts had conclusively proven
the causes of fat, we'd all be thin.

I have simply pulled together
scattered facts and synthesized them into
a viable, logical program, a program whose
very success testifies to its validity.

JUDY MAZEL

THE
BEVERLY
HILLS
DIET

I

A Diet for the Eighties

WELCOME TO THE WORLD OF THE GOLDEN PINEAPPLE

If you read this book carefully and understand and internalize the rules and the commandments, my diet will work for you. No one who's been committed to this program has failed to lose weight. When you become a Conscious Combiner, slimhood becomes a reality.

"Combiners" who participate in individual or group sessions give me much delightful and insightful feedback. Their enthusiasm helps nourish my program, reinforces its validity, and propels me to devote my life to its perpetuation and the abolition of the fat consciousness that pervades so many of my first-time clients.

"This is the first time in my whole life I've maintained. It's a miracle. I've always been up and down, up and down. . . . I've never been as disciplined as I have been on this diet." Or, as another new "Combiner" put it, "A lot of diets don't have hope, and this diet gives you hope. . . . It's a diet you can work with."

My clients number almost as many males as females and run

1

the gamut from teens to oldsters, from the obese to the slim main-tainer, from the high-powered executive to film stars to house-wives. Successful skinnies often reappear simply to lock back into that special support system the Beverly Hills Diet affords, to sing their new bodies' and, in tandem, my diet's praises.

"My energy has changed. There's no doubt about it." "As a thin person, I'm filled with self-respect and pride." "I've learned to rejoice in food and stay skinny." "I did it, and I'm totally in love with myself."

If you agree never to starve yourself and to stop thinking of potatoes and pasta as fattening, if going out of your way to find the ripest pineapples doesn't disturb you, if lobster and butter are more exciting than chicken without skin, if corn on the cob and artichokes have more appeal than cottage cheese and tomato slices, if popcorn sounds like more fun than carrot sticks, then the Beverly Hills Diet can work for you, too.

"I ordered pasta in a restaurant without guilt or shame. I ate as much as I wanted, and I didn't even have to sneak off of some-body else's plate." "My mother walked in and was horri-fied. . . . She asked me what I was doing. 'I'm eating my dinner,' I smugly replied. 'I'm allowed one pint of Haagen-Dazs ice cream.' "

You will learn that blowing it is a thing of the past because there is nothing out there you can't have. The trick is learning how and when to eat it and what to do to compensate for it. What to do to counter its effects, to make it digestible and thus nonfattening.

"I ate pizza and lived," exulted director John Calendo. "I had just finished the six-week Judy Mazel program, lost thirty-three pounds, and, frankly, looked better and felt better than I did in college. But then I had to go back to Chicago and direct my first play. I would be far from Judy's weekly menus, a born-again virgin stomach in a city where I would be prey to a gang of stocky, heavy-duty, deep-dish, Chicago-style pizzas. In L.A., I had even looked forward to watermelons, civilly eating them with a knife and fork, singling out the seeds as if they were gourmet delights! But those pizzas had come to symbolize Chicago and a period in my life that was as warm as the neighborhood restaurant where I ate them. Every fifth day in Chicago I would slowly, decorously and totally consume a *large* sausage, mushroom, double cheese pizza. *I didn't gain one pound.* Thank you, Judy."

You will learn to make every bite count. To experience food and make it an experience. To think about food when it doesn't count so you don't have to think about it when it does.

"I'm aware of everything I put in my mouth." "The way I was eating was crazed. I would wake up and, like many fat people, not feel hungry. Then about eleven or twelve in the morning I'd go and splurge. Now that I know I'm going to eat foods I really like, I can wait for them." "I get to eat anything I want as long as I plan for it."

You will understand and appreciate that food and wonderful restaurants, everything about eating that is important to you, *will be here tomorrow.* If you don't have it all now, you can have it later; if not later, then maybe tomorrow; *Nothing is leaving the planet.*

You will not only acknowledge your food fantasies, you will fulfill them. You're going to eat to your heart's content without eating your heart out. You are going to get away with murder without serving a life sentence.

I am *not* going to give you a strict diet with lists of foods you can't have. Rather, I am going to give you the tools to make slim-hood a forever reality. You will apply these tools to your own life-style, your own world, your own eating. Your diet will be a dream come true because it will include all the foods that have always caused you to break other diets. These foods are important to you, otherwise, you wouldn't have blown every other diet you've been on to eat them. Well, you won't have to blow this diet because it will be built around all your favorite foods.

You are about to experience a methodology combined with a philosophy, a way of relating to food that will ensure eternal slimhood. There is more to eating than meets the stomach, more to food than meets the mind.

Of course, no matter how effective my diet, you have to *care*. I can't *make* you lose weight and gain energy. *You* must do that. You have to embark on a love affair with yourself and with food. Begin today. Embrace and accept what you love so much. Let food work for you. You don't have to fight it anymore. It is no longer the enemy.

You have already taken that critical first step. If you didn't care, if you weren't motivated, you wouldn't have read this far, would you?

My hope is that my philosophy will enter your consciousness and alter it immeasurably and forever.

Remember, you don't have to be fat anymore, and you never have to be fat again.

What have you got to lose?

CONSCIOUS COMBINERS TELL ALL

Thousands are discovering the magic of the Beverly Hills Diet. Media around the country—*Mademoiselle, Vogue,* the *Los Angeles Times, Beverly Hills People,* the *Los Angeles Herald Examiner*—have featured Judy Mazel's diet discovery.

"Diet guru Judy Mazel takes Hollywood heavy-weights in hand and makes them svelte in a town where 'thin-is-in,'" trumpets the *New York Post.* "Eat your heart out" are words that celebrities as diverse as actress Sally Kellerman and singer Maria Muldaur have taken to their hearts, not their waistlines.

US refers to me as "uncanny." *Playgirl* featured a five-day Conscious Combining Plan, calling it a "beauty diet." Patrick Goldstein, in the *Los Angeles Reader*, spotlights me as "Hollywood's hottest diet guru." Susan Shultz, in *Phoenix Magazine*, says, "Judy Mazel has spawned the diet revolution of tomorrow." *New West* proclaims, ". . . the joy of [my] helping entertainers who have brought so much happiness to others."

The Chicago Sun-Times: "Look out Chicago! Judy Mazel, Hollywood's hottest midriff missionary . . . is headed the way of the cornfed Midwest. Mazel's hand-picked client's roster reads like an A-movie screening list."

Vogue, British Edition: "[Judy Mazel is a] new guru . . . whose training programme teaches that through informed food combining you can eat your way to permanent highs of physical and psychic energy."

Las Vegas Sun: "[Her] path turned out to be good nutrition. . . . Don't fret, you will be losing weight while you have your pint of chocolate ice cream. . . . It's not unusual for someone on Judy's diet to be seen eating lobster, pizza, chocolate cake, ice cream, or other foods usually considered diet no-nos."

Rona Barrett's Hollywood: "Everyone from "Dallas" 's Linda Gray to Washington's Jack Anderson has been sized up . . . by the "food combining" expert who says 'Let them eat cake. . . .' "

Because my diet works, it's fun, and it's livable, famous and highly visible persons, whose very livelihoods depend on their looks, energy, and slimhood, are becoming my disciples by the score.

"Judy's like a psychiatrist—she puts you in therapy," says Susan Haymer, producer for David Sheehan TV Specials. "It's not a diet. It's a fun way to eat."

"The bottom line, of course, is that it works. You lose weight," exults Pat Harrington, star of "One Day At A Time."

"I carried twenty extra pounds for twenty years. With Judy, I got it off. New foods, new tastes, it's just great!"

"Now I have a whole health consciousness," claims Claire, the fifteen-year-old daughter of film star Sally Kellerman. "I've lost thirty pounds—quickly and easily. I have energy . . . my skin is much nicer, clear and very soft. I have never felt better."

"Dallas" star Linda Gray was getting hypoglycemic from eating too many sweets on the set. She is one of many who are on my diet not to lose weight but to get healthy, to gain new energy. Says Linda, "I love not thinking about food, always knowing what I will be eating. It works perfectly into my busy schedule, and I thrive on munching cashews in my car."

In the *Los Angeles Herald Examiner*, Barbara Yaroslavsky, the wife of Los Angeles City Councilman, Zev Yaroslavsky, tells how we "make the necessary dietary adjustments" around her busy social and political schedules and attests to the success of my technique, noting that she's lost thirty-three pounds (ten in the first week) since beginning it. "I've made mistakes," she concedes. "But I've never *cheated*. I don't need to. I just ask for things and get them. I go to Victor Benish Bakery and eat an entire alligator coffee cake for lunch; it's one and a half feet long and eight inches wide, and it's filled with pecans—and I *still* lose weight," Barbara exclaims. "It's a totally different way of dieting, but so what? So life is different. Look, I think it's fantastic. And if I could convince my mother, it must be okay. She looks at me and can't believe her eyes."

Sally Kellerman, major film star, who makes fitness her number-one priority, expounds the virtues of my diet: "I've gone on many diets, but Judy's is the easiest. She has this instinct about what your body needs and an honesty you don't find in most nutritionists. When I start a picture, I'll call her up and say, 'Hey, Judy, I had this four-course meal last night, and I feel terrible—

what do I do?' and she'll come up with something inspired. Her diet is for the oral compulsive. . . ."

Recommending me to a business associate, George Sidney, a film director, explained, "She works around your likes and dislikes . . . and it all becomes a game. I'm sure she would relieve you of ten to twenty pounds in a few weeks. Believe me, it works. Give her a call. You'd be amazed how many people you know use her services. It's so easy. . . ."

As a former Miss America put it, "Of all the people selling skinny in the great metropolis of Beverly Hills (and I've met them all) I can honestly say that Judy Mazel is unique in that she is the only one who was as fat as an innertube and is now 102 pounds. That means to me that she went through the process herself and it works. . . . There is nothing you can say about the difficulty you're having in getting skinny that she has not experienced."

"As I continue 'out here' in the world," confides Carole Ita White, an actress featured in such TV shows as "Laverne & Shirley," I realize how important, how essential, the discipline of the program is to my life. It grounds me. It comforts me to have a plan and to stick to it. It affords me the opportunity to face my life and my needs. My life is not about dieting anymore. It is about functioning and surviving and earning a living in my art . . . and loving. Bless you Judy, and thanks."

Not only does the Beverly Hills Diet *work*, but it's also *fun*. Hollywood's stars—those most jaded to body fads—are singing its praises.

But what about the not-so-famous? What about those of us who share the agonies of dieting away from the bright spotlights, who again and again suffer the miseries and frustrations of broken diet promises, to whom losing weight and keeping it off is every bit as important as it is to the stars?

Dear Judy,

I can no longer contain my delight in view of the wonderful results obtained from your diet.

I want to acknowledge the contribution you have made to my life and my body.

I have never felt better emotionally or physically.

The approach is medically sound and viable.

This is a great solution for compulsive overeating; at last I can live to eat and not get fat over it. Bravo Judy, and thanks!

                                        Marvin B. Meisler, D.D.S.

Says Loree Frazier, "I am happy to announce that not only am I fifteen pounds lighter, but I have not felt so well and so vibrant in many a year, which is a beautiful plus. My friends say the transformation is like a miracle. B.J. (before Judy), not only was I overweight, but I also suffered constantly from stomach upsets and very sluggish elimination. I was told my gall bladder was barely functioning. Thanks to your help, those days are gone forever.

"With what you've taught me about food and how it relates to my body, I feel totally alive and totally satisfied. I thank you not only for myself but for the many others who, hopefully, will have the good fortune to meet you."

Bonnie Pick, law student, says:

"Anyone who could get me off sugar, salt, and junk food *and* make me feel and look as good as I do deserves tons of credit."

"Judy Mazel and her fabulous food philosophy entered my life and turned me into a veritable nymphette," says publicist Carol Green.

Las Vegas socialite Estee Rousso inscribes, "Dearest Judy—I surrender to you that aspect of me that needs to be taught the relationship between energy and food. . . ."

"You have changed me and my life so radically in the past

months. . . . I love you and thank you," writes New Yorker Peggy Pierrepont.

I have changed their lives and, if you'll let me, I'll change your life, too.

Can you imagine what it will be like to look forward to getting on the scale? Can you guess what it will be like to look at yourself in the mirror and see the body you always fantasized having? Can you imagine never being fat again? Ever?

Hard, isn't it, when you have been on so many diets and failed on so many diets. How many pounds have you lost in your life? And then regained? Are you ready to lose them forever?

If you are sick of diets and dieting, if you are prepared to begin thinking about food, learning about food and yourself, if you are willing to make conscious choices, then the Beverly Hills Diet will work for you, too.

II

The Transformation of a Food Junkie

FAT, FATTER, FATTEST: THE WRETCHED TREADMILL

All my life I have loved to eat and lived to eat. I still do. I can match you or anyone, food fantasy for food fantasy, bite for bite. I can sit down and luxuriate in a rack of lamb for two—without leaving a shred on my plate—a whole Long Island duckling, an eighteen-ounce steak, a triple order of linguini, or an entire cheesecake. When food is in my mouth, I'm in an altered state of consciousness. My heart sings and my soul soars. I never have enough. I'm totally absorbed. Somehow, I never get full. I never get tired of eating.

Yet for the last six years, my five-feet-four-inch frame has not varied more than three pounds from my ideal weight of 102. I eagerly look forward to getting on my scale every morning, to ferreting out the tiniest bikinis to wear on the beach. I'm not afraid to layer on the bulkiest clothes when I'm in snow country —and I owe it all to a way of eating that I devised and developed —a methodology and a philosophy that has become the Beverly Hills Diet.

It wasn't always that way. Far from it. I began life as a skinny.

But suddenly, at the age of eight, I started to gain weight. I vividly remember being taken to a "diet doctor," who gave me my first diet pills. From that moment on my life seesawed between fat and chubby; I was hooked into a maze of diet doctors, shots, pills, thyroid pills, supplements, laxatives, diets, diets, and more diets.

Everybody watched what I ate. And what I ate, in turn, occupied more and more of my energy and my life. I loved to clear the table because that was my chance to grab everybody's leftovers. My family constantly nagged, "Are you still eating, Judy? Haven't you had enough?" The more they hounded me, the more I wanted to eat.

When I graduated from grammar school, my mother was shocked because I was too fat to fit into children's clothes. She had to take me to an adult-clothing store—and pay adult prices—for my graduation dress.

When I was fourteen and had swelled to 145 pounds, I decided for myself to go on a diet. My pills were increased. My nerves throbbed and my head ached. Insomnia became a fixation. I was a real brat. But I stuck to it and dropped to 114 pounds.

Within a month, I'd gained back every pound. And back I went to the diet doctor's office, squeezed in the waiting room among all the other fatties, feeling hostile and miserable. At home I was getting mixed messages: "I love you, but you're fat. If you're fat, I won't love you."

I used to sneak money out of my mother's wallet so I'd have money for a pizza when I stayed home alone on Saturday nights. I'd hide the smelly wrappings under my bed and guiltily slip them into a neighbor's garbage can when I thought no one was looking. Of course, whether by intention or not, I was always getting caught.

I hovered between a size fourteen and sixteen, chunky but

not grossly obese. By the end of high school I was on everything: thyroid pills, diet pills, laxatives.

College was more of the same except that boys became an important—and conspicuously absent—part of my life. I became the consumate performer, anything to compensate for being fat. And I knew, no matter what else anybody said about me, good or bad, he or she could always add "and she's fat!"

In desperation, I went to the ultimate diet doctor in Chicago. He put me on the most high-powered dosage of diet pills I'd ever been on and added something new, diuretics. For the second time in my life I became almost thin—130 pounds. But I never really felt thin. In addition, the side effects of the pills and diuretics I'd been piling into my body were beginning to take a toll on my system.

When I finally felt socially acceptable, I decided to study acting, and I moved to L.A. With massive effort, I kept my weight down. In order to maintain that weight, I pumped up my dosage of thyroid pills, diuretics, and an uncountable number of diet pills a day. My insomnia and headaches hounded me with a vengeance. I'd awaken in the morning, take a diet pill, get back into bed, and wait for it to take effect.

I knew that what I was doing wasn't right, that spending sixty dollars a month at the pharmacy wasn't normal, that I was killing myself, but I didn't know what to do, which way to turn. The health revolution had started, but I thought the people who shopped in health-food stores and didn't eat meat were weirdos and hippies. Nutrition was a word I had heard in school and the meaning of which I didn't really know. It means, by the way, the role food plays in the health of the human body. It never oc- curred to me that what I was eating and the pills I was taking were causing and perpetuating my problems, that it was my Chinese dinners that Chairman Mao could have attended or the potato chips I imported by the case from Chicago. I only knew that if I cut back, even ever so slightly, on the pills I was taking, if, God forbid, I should find myself away from home overnight without my *Lasix*, I would blow up like a balloon. I gained and lost eight to ten pounds each day.

Finally, I convinced a doctor in Los Angeles to put me in the hospital for tests. In ten days, off my drugs, I gained twenty-two pounds. My legs bloated, my eyes puffed into slits.

The doctors pronounced my thyroid as nonfunctional and my adrenal and pituitary glands as virtually useless. They decided they couldn't take me off the drugs, and I resigned myself to going through life half fat, more or less drugged, and miserable.

KICKING THE HABIT

On a ski trip six months later, I slammed into a tree on my first run and was knocked unconscious. I woke up in the hospital with a broken leg. It was then that I experienced something new in my life, something besides a broken leg: I started experiencing the world from a new vantage point. Lying in the hospital, helpless, feeling my leg, I became aware of my body as an entity, a synergy of its parts—each dependent on the other. As my leg mended, I began to understand and accept the fact that my body was a product of what fueled it—the food that energized it and the drugs that sapped it. I wanted to know more.

I began devouring books on nutrition, reaching out for anything that would feed my new hunger for nutritional knowledge. One day, in the midst of my studies, it really hit me: Hey! I could be healthy. I could really be whole—without the pills, the diuretics, the thyroid pills, the headaches, and the insomnia. Without the doctors, the hospitals, the misery, and the self-hate. I was obsessed with getting healthy—and thin.

When my leg healed, I stepped up my studies. I haunted health-food stores. I sought out doctors, scientists, nutritionists.

I spent six months in Santa Fe studying under the famed nutritionist Scott Gershen, president of the Sonta College of Natural Medicine. I trusted him because he had a strong background in medicine. And he made sense. He wasn't one of those healers who talks a good game but doesn't know the basics of science. I was suspicious of hypes, of kooks, of health nuts, of people trumpeting messages of their internal messiahs.

I learned that there were healthful equivalents of the junk foods I adored. It didn't involve sacrifice. Not that I would *ever* deprive myself, even then. I started reading labels, studying how food manufacturers processed their products. I continued to upgrade the quality of the food I was eating.

Slowly, I began throwing away my pills—without swelling up, without gaining weight. In fact, I lost weight. I began to discover the way a person ought to feel. Gradually I edged over the line toward health.

Now I was really motivated to change. I wanted to drop my "fat consciousness" once and for all, to become skinny once and for all. From my studies and internship in Santa Fe, I'd learned about the workings of the body and nutritional needs. Still, I needed to know more.

I started studying myself and observing that cavernous disparity, that split, between mind and body. I acknowledged my inability to feel my body. Somehow it had never occurred to me that it's my head that tells my body what to do; I had always thought my feet were too far from my brain to have any control over them. I began to heal that split through various forms of body therapy: Reichian Therapy, Rolfing, the Alexander Technique, Dance Therapy, Vocal Bio Matrix, Bio Energetics—you name it, I tried it. I internalized the fact that my body really is a synergy of its parts, that it really does depend, in every way, on what I put into it for what it puts out. I was breaking down my armor, getting in touch with my body and actually feeling it—

just as I had when I had broken my leg. I was off the diuretics and thyroid pills, and I didn't gain weight or bloat. The cycle was destroyed. I went from 122 pounds to 116 pounds. But I still felt fat. I still had at least 10 more pounds to lose.

I realized that all my dietary beliefs, my acceptance of what scores of diet doctors had told me, everything I had grown up believing about food, eating, and fat was . . . *suspect.* Maybe the answers really weren't out there yet. I knew I couldn't go on any of the old diets again. Not only did they not work, they were not healthy!

I was seeking the ultimate diet. Nothing I tried really worked. Stillman; Atkins; counting carbs, calories; eating my dinner for breakfast. All were rigid prescriptions for failure.

I was running out of books to read and nutritionists to learn from. One day when I was wondering whether there ever *would* be an answer, I pulled off the freeway in search of cashews and discovered the missing link in a health-food store—the catalyst that propelled me to develop the Beverly Hills Diet. What I found was a book about enzymes and the digestive system. The author suggested that the combination of foods eaten was the key to good digestion, and I immediately zeroed in on this as the key to losing fat. I began reading about enzymes and the pivotal role they play in the digestive process. I hit the libraries and read everything I could get my hands on about those little devils.

As I discovered the basic laws of digestion and the role enzymes play in food processing, I began to throw out everything I had been taught to believe about a balanced meal. I realized that while it is true we need the proper balance of protein, carbohydrates, and fats in our diet, the idea of eating a "balanced" meal is as absurd as wearing two skirts or two pairs of shoes at the same time.

And I threw out everything my fat self had always believed about diets and dieting. Prehistoric man didn't eat a balanced diet. He ate some berries; he'd kill an animal and eat it. He'd find some nuts and a few slugs. Somewhere in the course of our social evolution it became "convenient" to eat breakfast, lunch, and dinner. "Convenient" to eat a "balanced" meal. But was "balanced" in fact a true description of what our diet should be? Was "balanced" based on the facts of health?

I began to understand that there is no food that is intrinsically good or bad; it's what we eat those foods *with* that has potential instead. Being fat has little to do with what you eat or how much you eat but rather the combinations of the foods you eat. The key is digestion. As long as food is fully digested, fully processed through the body, you will not gain weight. It's only undigested food, food that is "stuck" in your body, for whatever reason, that accumulates and becomes fat.

I began developing a system of eating based on enzymatic laws. There were no rules, nothing to go by except the facts to be gathered from widely disparate sources and applied together, synthesized, and tested. What better subject than myself? I began building a process by experimenting on myself.

I first experimented just with the "good" foods, the "diet" foods I knew would work—lean meat, skinless chicken, cottage cheese, and broiled fish. Of course they worked. But to make this a day-to-day reality for me, I knew I had to include all the foods I loved, all the foods I had previously blown my diet for. I knew myself well enough to realize I could only stick to a controlled regimen for so long. Here's where it got tricky.

The other diets were all the same, give or take a few celery sticks. Each dictated no bread, no pasta, no potatoes, no sweets. Well, big deal! No wonder they worked. But forever?

I know I'm an emotional eater. If I weren't, if I could stay on a controlled food intake, then all those other diets would have worked for me. But I eat in response to a feeling. And I can't stop those feelings from happening. Have you noticed that virtually every "eater" you know has been described as "sensitive"?

I knew I wasn't going to stop eating, that food was urgently important to me. The problem was that food hadn't been working *for* me, and I had learned how vital that was. I had to make it work.

I still had that old diet consciousness, which dictated that the only way I could give myself permission to blow my diet was by telling myself that tomorrow I'd go back on it. It was inconceivable to me that I could be on anything other than a strictly controlled eating regimen and not mushroom to three hundred pounds.

But everything I was reading and studying, everything I was pulling together, was telling me otherwise. I had to try.

I had to create a diet that would be a permanent way of life, a diet that would include every food I'd craved during all those miserable years growing up. Surely enzymes were the key. Fattening had to mean something more than calories. Calories, I had learned, simply represented energy. My research on enzymes made me realize that fattening had to do with indigestibility. How well our body processes the food we eat and how those foods get clogged in our systems.

I began eating one food at a time, having discovered that most enzymes can't work simultaneously and that many cancel one another out in our digestive systems. I also discovered that if I didn't have too many foods, tastes, or textures at once, I was less likely to overeat. I like to compare the mouth of an eater to the keys of a finely tuned piano, each bite ringing out a different note. The harmony goes on—the tune is endless.

I got up my courage and began experimenting with bread, nuts, potatoes—the not-so-safe foods. Then I tried the foods I'd always broken my diets for: pasta, pancakes, and finally ice cream and desserts. Eureka! It was working! By eating a single food at a time, I was working with my digestive process . . . and not gaining weight. I still couldn't eat real salty foods without bloating, but I discovered that foods containing small amounts of salt didn't necessarily spell disaster.

My experiments intensified. I learned that tropical fruits have an incredibly high concentration of digestive enzymes. Was it possible that the enzymes in these fruits could make hard-to-digest foods less fattening? Could their enzymatic capabilities be used to offset the indigestibility of fattening mixed foods?

I tried it. I'd never tasted a mango in my life. I had no idea what a papaya looked like. Are you kidding? A steak and ribs and pizza freak? I concentrated on which enzymes would counteract which food groups. I tested and tried and ate . . . and ate . . . and ate. And still I lost weight. I was obviously on to something fabulous!

For eight months I matched enzyme against enzyme, learning to literally "have my cake and eat it too." I began to accept the fact that slimhood could be a reality. That once I got there, I could stay there. That all I had to give up were a few old neuroses, a few worn beliefs that had to do with balanced meals, and a few pounds. I concentrated on health and on maximizing the nutritional value of my diet. I set out a program for myself that was initially to maintain, not lose, weight. But I continued to lose. I began scheduling my favorite foods rather than eating them so compulsively, and then I followed them with the proper counteracting enzyme.

EUREKA! CONSCIOUS COMBINING DISCOVERED

My weight dropped to ninety-seven pounds. I was dealing with the world from an entirely different perspective. I loved it!

I began to love me! I stopped being scared. I knew I would never be fat again. I could eat anything I wanted.

Throughout my testing, my experimenting, and my intense excitement at having discovered the key to my happiness, I kept in mind the emotional side of my eating. I know those trite expressions were filled with truth: swallowing your anger, swallowing your pride, starved for attention, starved for affection, eating your heart out—all those expressions applied to me.

I knew no matter what kind of methodology I had devised, when it came to eating, I was always going to be responding to my feelings with my mouth. To this day when I experience a certain type of disappointment I crave spareribs. I knew my methodology had to allow for those emotional moments.

I found that I didn't have to be 100 percent disciplined, that I didn't always have to plan for what I wanted to eat, that I could give in to the spontaneity of the moment because I had locked on to the corrective counterparts for my indulgences. I could give myself permission to indulge because blowing it didn't mean a tomorrow of nevers. I didn't have to make every meal the "last supper." I didn't have to experience a "fear of eating."

The diet I had made for myself answered all my prayers— a dream come true. What I chose to eat determined what I had to eat because my diet was nothing more than following a series of simple rules, and following them the day after a splurge was easy.

By this time I was scheduling myself day by day, so that one day determined the next, each day hinged on the day before and the day after. I continued to study the enzymatic capabilities of different foods and how they affect digestibility and fat. Success followed success. It got so I could accurately predict the effects *before* experimenting. I was rarely wrong. It became a matter of streamlining, pushing the limit, adding neutrals (fruits without enzymatic capabilities) for interest, seeking out fat and thin friends and applying my methodology to their diets. More and more I became acutely aware of how I was feeling, aware of the tremendous new energy reserves I had. I was determined to build that energy into my diet forever.

My metamorphosis did not go unnoticed. Friends began asking for help, and I began responding. I decided to devote myself to the Conscious Combining of foods, health, and slimhood. After all, I had acquired and developed this special knowledge, and I felt an obligation to share it with anyone who had a weight problem.

SLIMHOOD FOREVER: HAVING MY CAKE AND EATING IT TOO

I worked out different programs, which concentrated primarily on fruit, for some close friends. They lost weight dramatically. Word spread from L.A. to Las Vegas to Chicago to Phoenix. People were learning there was, at last, hope for the hopeless. Converts mushroomed. Hollywood, the jet set, the world famous began clamoring for my secrets. Doctors and psychiatrists began recommending me to their overweight patients. Southern California's elite swarmed at my door—and went away skinny. The Beverly Hills Diet became a reality.

Most of my clients can afford to go anywhere in the world, tap any resource, luxuriate at any spa, yet they come to me because they know my diet works.

In response to demand, I have written this book so you can share in the success of my method. For more than six years I have stayed within three pounds of my ideal weight. I cannot expect you to understand the happiness and rewards this has brought me—at least not yet. Only by experiencing Conscious Combining through the Beverly Hills Diet can you appreciate what eternal slimhood really means. I have changed the lives of hundreds of former fatties. I will change your life too.

If we can do it, so can you.

III

Conscious Combining
Explained

HOW FOOD BECOMES YOU

I am not concerned with what you eat or even how much you eat. What matters is *when* you eat and, most important, what you eat it *with*. I repeat, diet does not mean deprivation. It means a way of life.

You can have your cake and eat it too—if you eat it one piece at a time. That's what the Beverly Hills Diet is all about.

To intellectually justify this new approach to eating you must understand it. I'm not going to take your heart out of your stomach, but I'm going to put your head in. You need to understand how food becomes you. Only then can you experience food in its truest sense. Only then can you become aware of your body as a synergy of its parts, each dependent on the other, each dependent for its very life on the food, the fuel, you give it.

In simplest terms, fat means indigestion, or undigested food. Undigested food means fat. When your body doesn't process food, doesn't digest it, that food turns into fat.

Essentially, your body takes the food you give it and turns it into nutrients, "body food." A nutrient is a substance needed by living organisms to maintain life, health, and the reproductive

21

processes. The nutrients are vitamins, minerals, amino acids, glucose, lipids, and water.

Digestion, or the breakdown of food into nutrients, is done by enzymes, little chemical reactors that are in the food we eat or are promoted and made in our bodies by the food we eat. Basically, different enzymes work on the three different food groups—proteins, carbohydrates, and fats.

Each food group has its own set of enzymes. Generally, a protein enzyme can work only on proteins, a carbohydrate enzyme can work only on carbohydrates, and a fat enzyme can work only on fats.

Not only can the enzymes not cross over into other food groups, but they are often antagonistic toward one another, and the presence of one can actually prevent another from doing its work. Enzymes are very particular substances, and while there are hundreds there are only three you need to know about:

PTYALIN   The enzyme essential for digesting carbohydrates. It appears in our saliva and is activated when we chew.

HYDROCHLORIC ACID   This is technically not an enzyme but its function is much the same. It is in our stomachs and is responsible for the digestion of fat.

PEPSIN   To be broken down into nutrients our bodies can use, proteins require two enzymes: pepsin and hydrochloric acid. Pepsin appears in our stomachs.

To know how food becomes you, we need to go a few steps further and understand how these enzymes work. This explains why digestibility is the key. The digestive process is the process whereby our bodies take food and turn it into nutrients so we can use it, so it can become body food, so that the process of life can continue.

The body processes food in four stages: digestion, absorption, metabolism, and elimination.

Digestion:
Stage One of the Digestive Process

During the first stage, food is turned into nutrients by three parts of the body: the mouth, the stomach, and the small intestine.

THE MOUTH   Eating a carbohydrate activates the enzyme ptyalin, which breaks the carbohydrate down into nutrients. Other foods—proteins, fats, and that special category of carbohydrates, fruit, are not affected by this enzyme and pass through the mouth into the stomach.

THE STOMACH   When a carbohydrate reaches your stomach, if it has been properly digested, it is in the form of maltose, a crystalline sugar. Your stomach breaks down the maltose even further and sends it on its way.

If food is a protein, it will be broken down by the enzyme pepsin, which is activated by hydrochloric acid. First it will get a hydrochloric-acid shower to cut through the fat and break it up. At this point the pepsin is activated to soften and break up the protein into amino acids. After these two steps, the hydrochloric acid and pepsin work together to further digest protein foods into amino acids.

When fat enters your stomach, your body uses hydrochloric acid, as well as other substances, to break it up into lipids, fat's special nutrient form.

THE SMALL INTESTINE   Food is then sent to the small intestine. In your small intestine are millions of little villi eagerly waiting to absorb your now usable nutrients so that they can be transported to all your hungry cells. With the exception of fruit, by the time food reaches the small intestine it has already been broken down into nutrients. Fruit becomes a nutrient within the small intestine.

A note about fruit. While all other foods have to spend time digesting in your mouth and/or your stomach, fruit is an exception because it contains all the enzymes it needs to form nutrients within itself; so your body's enzymes are not required either in your mouth or in your stomach to process it, and the fruit slips through, barely hesitating. Although the stomach doesn't call up enzymes to act on the fruit, it does rot and ripen it so it can slide through to the small intestines. This occurs so quickly that, before you can even finish eating a pineapple, your first bites are being turned into nutrients in your small intestines and are already being transported into your bloodstream.

Absorption:
Stage Two of the Digestive Process

This is the process whereby all your little cells are nourished. Broken-down nutrients are transported to your cells, which lap them up from your bloodstream and put them to work. This is also the stage when all water-soluble vitamins and minerals are absorbed into the bloodstream.

Metabolism:
Stage Three of the Digestive Process

This is the point at which all those digested nutrients are converted into building materials. This is the payoff, the process that creates your flesh and blood, that generates your energy. This is the stage at which you feel what you eat, where the quality of the food you eat makes a difference. The most common complaint I get from my clients is "I have a slow metabolism." Your body, like an automobile, can only run on the fuel it's fed. If you put a low-grade gasoline in a Rolls-Royce, it will soon need to be towed. If the food that fuels you is of low quality, your body will not function optimally.

Elimination:
The Final Stage of the Digestive Process

Whatever nutrients your body doesn't need are eliminated through the mouth by breathing, through the skin when you perspire, and, most important, through excretion by urination and bowel movements. Excretion is the most active form of elimination.

If any one of the four steps of food processing (the digestive process) is faulty or weak, all are affected. A chain reaction takes place. The result? Indigestion. You may not even be aware of it, or you may accept it as inevitable. The obvious symptoms? Gas, heartburn, or a stomachache. The not-so-obvious? Insomnia, depression, headaches, lack of energy, nervous tension, and dull skin and hair. The most overlooked yet most obvious of all symptoms of indigestion is *fat*. Well, why not? Fat, after all, is food or something that has been ingested—artificial sweeteners, preservatives, diet sodas—anything that has been ingested that has not been digested, absorbed, metabolized, or eliminated.

Fat indicates that somewhere along the line the digestive process has fouled up. For most fat people, the problem does not occur during stages two or three, absorption or metabolism. Although we'd all like to think we have a slow metabolism, sorry, it's not so. In fact, it's the rarest exception.

Occasionally there is difficulty with elimination, perhaps because your food is too low in fiber, it's over-refined which causes mucus and pits (small holes) in your intestines. This, in turn, impedes elasticity and slows down elimination.

The problem is usually in the first stage—digestion—when food is turned into nutrients. If we foul up in this stage, our bodies don't have a chance. It's this stage that we focus on in the Conscious Combining Technique, the key to the Beverly Hills Diet.

If our enzymatic system is functioning as it should, odds are that the second, third, and fourth stages are humming happily along. But if food isn't broken down into nutrients, it can't be absorbed. If it can't be absorbed, it can't be metabolized. If it can't be metabolized, it can't be used or eliminated. If it can't be used or eliminated, it gets stuck in your body—*and turns into fat!*

Remember, fat is nothing more than food or something you have ingested that has not been digested. If it had been properly processed, it would have gone through all four steps and it wouldn't still be there. Make sense?

Nutrients: The Nub of It All

Moving right along. . . . What are these nutrients? Why are they so important? How do they manipulate the fat equation?

Nutrients are essential for the creation and maintenance of life. They are what we are made of. They are in the food we eat, and they contain chemical substances that provide energy and generate growth. They repair our body tissues and promote body processes. Our very being depends on nutrients. Our bodies are nothing more than flesh and blood and energy. If we could be broken down and put in a test tube, we would be nothing more than a combination of six nutrients: vitamins, minerals, amino acids, glucose, lipids, and water.

Vitamins perform specific and vital functions in the ongoing process of life. They carry on the process of life. They are organic substances absolutely essential for growth and health. They contain enzymes and aid in building our major body structures. Examples are vitamins C, B, A, and D.

Minerals can be either organic or inorganic, and they exist in our bones, teeth, tissue, muscle, blood, and nerve cells. They affect processes such as hormonal production, muscle response, nervous-system communication, and fluid balances, plus of course much more. Examples are calcium, chlorine, iron, potassium, sulfur, phosphorous, and magnesium.

Amino Acids are the nutrients derived from protein. They provide our body with its flesh and blood. They are the body's building blocks. Amino acids build our muscles, blood, skin, hair and nails, and even our internal organs, such as the heart and the brain.

Amino acids are highly versatile. After completing their role as building blocks, they have the potential of going one step further and becoming glucose, the blood sugar that provides energy. You'll remember that amino acids wind up in your bloodstream to be used as the body's building blocks. Once the body has decided it's had enough, it turns the leftovers into glucose. Amino acids are the only nutrient that can perform two functions. They become both body builders and, much later, energy. This energy is inefficient because it's slow and unpredictable, therefore inferior.

Before your body turns back the amino acids so they can be transformed into glucose, it makes sure that each and every cell has had its fill. If you've got a big body, it's going to keep each and every little cell fed and nourished to maintain your size. When you lose weight, those cells are not eliminated. They simply shrink, ever-poised to plump back up into fat.

The energy that is derived from protein at the end of that process is, by necessity, diluted. Think about it. When was the last time you had high energy on a high-protein diet? You see, the protein stays in your stomach anywhere from four to twelve hours, undergoing twelve digestive steps, and only then is it absorbed into your bloodstream. First your body picks and chooses what it needs to replenish itself and does so. Then the amino acids are reshuffled and used.

Glucose is the gasoline we run on. It keeps our hearts beating, our blood flowing. It lets us shrug our shoulders and put one foot in front of the other. It is the only nutrient that becomes instant energy.

The way we are meant to get glucose is from glucose-containing foods, which means carbohydrates. They provide glucose immediately, as soon as they are metabolized. Carbohydrates turn into energy. That's their purpose. Because this is a high-energy diet, the Beverly Hills Diet is a high-carbohydrate diet.

We're all locked into thinking that carbohydrates are more fattening than protein. Yet both protein and carbohydrates have the same number of calories—four—for each gram of weight. There is *no* caloric difference between the two.

Calories are energy, pure and simple. Carbohydrates are energy, pure and simple. Remember, glucose is energy and carbohydrates turn into glucose. You should get your energy from carbohydrates because that is what they are meant to provide. It is far more efficient than getting your energy from protein. Getting energy from protein is a waste because, remember, protein only becomes energy (that is to say, amino acids only become glucose) after it has completed the building process. Consider all that extra energy you use in the process of converting protein to energy. All that wasted time before you get it and utilize it.

Lipids are the stored energy contained in fats. Our reserve bank. The most concentrated source of energy in our diets. One gram of fat yields about nine calories versus the four in a gram of carbohydrate or protein. Lipids also act as carriers for the fat-soluble vitamins, A, E, D, and K. Without the proper balance of usable fats in our diet, our bodies can't assimilate or use these vitamins. Lipids protect our organs and insulate our bodies. Lipids are to fat what glucose is to carbohydrates and amino acids are to protein.

Water is what holds it all together. More than two thirds of your body weight is water. It's the essential constituent of your cells; it's what keeps it all going and flowing; it's what keeps all the other nutrients happy inside your little cells. Water maintains balance and harmony. It's responsible for and involved in nearly every body process, including digestion, absorption, circulation, and excretion. Water is necessary for all your body's building functions, and it helps maintain a normal body temperature and is vital in carrying waste materials out of your body.

An adult body typically holds forty-five quarts of water at any one time and loses approximately three quarts a day, although this fluctuates from one to more than ten, depending on your activity and environment.

Not surprisingly, some foods are about 80 percent water. Fruits and vegetables in particular.

Protein foods are the exception—they are the only ones that don't contain a great deal of water. This is one reason you have to drink a lot of water when you're on a high-protein diet. Yet digesting protein foods requires huge stores of water. To quench its thirst, protein sucks water out of your cells. That's why when you go off your high-protein diet, you're likely to regain much of the weight you lost. Your cells are desperate to replenish their lost liquid, and they do so the moment carbohydrates are reintroduced into your body. They lap up enough carbohydrates, naturally high in water, to eliminate their deficit, and in the process you regain the weight you lost—the weight that was, in fact, little more than liquids that were appropriated from your poor, parched cells. No wonder losers on high-protein diets often have that taut and haggard look! Something you won't get on the Beverly Hills Diet. In fact, many of my Combiners are accused of having had face-lifts.

When thinking about nutrients, remember that each has a

specific role to play. *None* can be duplicated. *Each* is critical to our very existence. Vitamins and minerals carry on the process of life. Amino acids build our flesh and blood. Glucose and lipids provide our energy, immediate and reserve. Water is what holds it all together and maintains balance and harmony. We're like a machine. Gasoline does one thing, oil another, water still another. Without fuel, the machine stops. Without essential nutrients, our bodies stop.

FOOD GROUPS—
THE WHO, WHAT, WHERE, AND HOW

To make food really work for you and to understand why it often works against you, in this streamlined, super-efficient fast food world of ours, you need to be aware of what kinds of foods exist and which groups they belong to, so you can accurately predict the enzymatic action they invoke.

You have learned that there are three major food groups: *proteins, carbohydrates,* and *fats.* There is also a special subcategory: *legumes.*

Legumes are special because they are half protein and half carbohydrate.

It is the proper balance of these three food groups that maintains a healthy, slim, and well-functioning body. All foods contain one or more of these nutrients. Most foods contain *all* of them, some protein, some carbohydrate, and some fat. Proteins, are more prevalent than you might suspect. Even a watermelon, for example, very obviously a carbohydrate, contains 25 percent protein. The classification of foods is determined by breaking them down to their nutrient components and determining the major component.

If a food is at least 51 percent amino acids, it is classified as a protein. If it is at least 51 percent glucose, it is considered a carbohydrate, and if it is at least 51 percent lipids, it qualifies as a fat.

Virtually all experts agree that the largest percentage of your calories should come from carbohydrates. If you work out a calorie breakdown, it should look like this: 50 percent carbohydrates, 30 percent fats, and 20 percent proteins.

On to the food groups:

Proteins

ANIMAL PROTEINS	ANIMAL PROTEINS (*Cont.*)
Beef	Lamb
Fish	Pork
Fowl	Eggs

DAIRY PROTEINS	DAIRY PROTEINS (*Cont.*)
Milk	Ice cream
Cheese	Cheesecake
Yogurt	

NUT PROTEINS	NUT PROTEINS (*Cont.*)
Nuts	Avocado
Seeds	

Fats

Butter	Cream, sour and heavy
Oil	

Carbohydrates

FRUITS	FRUITS (*Cont.*)
All fruits	Brandy
Champagne	Cognac
Wine	

MINI CARBS
Herbs
Asparagus
Celery
Crookneck squash
Kale
Lettuce
Mushrooms

MINI CARBS (*Cont.*)
Mustard greens
Parsley
Spinach
Summer squash
Swiss chard
Watercress
Zucchini

MIDI CARBS
Beets
Broccoli
Brussel sprouts
Cabbage
Carrots
Cauliflower
Cucumbers
Eggplant
Leeks

MIDI CARBS (*Cont.*)
Onions
Parsnips
Peas
Peppers (green, red, and chile)
Radishes
Shallots
String beans
Tomatoes
Turnips

MAXI CARBS
Artichokes
Breads
Buckwheat
Bulgar
Cake
Chocolate
Cookies
Corn
Grains
Liquors, all distilled (*see*
   Glossary)

MAXI CARBS (*Cont.*)
Millet
Pasta
Popcorn
Potatoes
Rice
Winter squash
All desserts, except those made
   with cheese

The ordering of the carbs is fixed by their molecular structure and their complexity, with maxi carbs being the most com-

plex. The more complex, the more enzymatic action necessary to digest it. And, thus, the longer the digestion time.

Don't be afraid of the maxi carbs. They give you the most energy. Remember, *nothing* is fattening by itself.

Legumes

Lentils	Pinto beans
Soybeans	Lima beans
Garbanzo beans	Kidney beans
Peanuts	

ENZYMES IN ACTION

Now that you know about nutrients and food groups and the role enzymes play in digestion and fat, we can look at enzymes in action. Here is the heart of the Beverly Hills Diet and its technique. This is where it all falls into place. Are you still with me? Hang on just a little longer. It will be well worth it!

How to Turn Carbohydrates into an Enemy

Carbs digest in your mouth through the work of the enzyme ptyalin, which is secreted in your saliva when you chew. If a carb hits your stomach without being in the form of maltose (via the action of ptyalin in your mouth), your stomach becomes frustrated and says, "What am I going to do with you? I don't have any ptyalin to digest you!"

And here the carb stays and stays, festering, fermenting, and rotting—not properly digesting—and ultimately turning into FAT.

There are three things that will neutralize ptyalin and make carbs indigestible:

1. *If you don't chew.* When your mother told you as a child to chew your food, she may not have known why, but she was right.

If you don't chomp that noodle, if you don't feel the sensual pleasure of a baked potato in your mouth, if you don't crunch your popcorn or luxuriate in the taste of fresh sourdough bread, if you just let that delectable food slide down your throat, then it will be fattening. You haven't triggered the ptyalin.

2. *Adding sweeteners.* It's not the pancake that's fattening. It's the syrup on top of the pancake that makes you gain weight. It's not the bread that's fattening, it's not the butter, it's the sweetener in that bread. It's the combination of a sweetener and the carb that's devastating.

It's the sweet in a sweet roll that makes it a killer. Any time you add a sweetener—and that means sugar, honey, maple syrup, molasses, or even raisin syrup—to a maxi carb, it's *no go.* The combination of a sweetener and a maxi carb neutralizes the enzyme pytalin. Pancakes drenched with butter—terrific. Add a single drop of syrup? Sorry.

3. *Mixing protein and carbohydrates* is equally destructive. When a fat-containing protein food hits your stomach, it activates those two enzymes, hydrochloric acid first and later pepsin. Hydrochloric acid breaks up any fat in the food and also activates the pepsin so it can break down the protein. When the hydrochloric acid and pepsin begin functioning simultaneously, the two enzymes set up an acid medium that neutralizes the carbohydrate enzyme, pytalin. In other words, ptyalin, the carb-digesting enzyme, is shut off as soon as hydrochloric acid and pepsin are working together.

The digestion of protein is so slow and unpredictable that, in terms of pounds gained or lost, once you have eaten a protein in the course of the day, there is no way your body can then digest a carbohydrate—not so much as a mushroom, a brussel sprout, or a piece of bread.

Meat remains in a particularly efficient stomach for about

eight to ten hours, poultry for about seven hours, and fish for approximately six hours. Keep in mind that most of us, having been on such high-protein, high-fat diets have pitifully inefficient stomachs.

All is not lost, however. Through time and the great resiliency of your body and with the help of this process you are about to begin, the efficiency of your stomach will increase significantly.

Clocking Your Enzymes to Unlock the Secrets of Combining

Protein foods are the hardest to digest because they require triple enzymatic action—hydrochloric acid, then pepsin, and then the two in combination; because of this they spend the most time in your stomach. Most proteins require twelve full steps before they are thoroughly digested.

Dairy products are by far the toughest protein foods to digest. Their high-fat and low-moisture content suppresses the very enzyme they need for digestion, hydrochloric acid, and a great struggle takes place in your stomach. We've all heard that drinking milk coats your stomach. True. But why would you want to coat your stomach when you want to digest something? By coating your stomach you're suppressing the very enzymes you need for digestion.

Carbs. The more complex the carbohydrate, the longer it will be in your stomach being digested. Maxi carbs are more complex than midi carbs, which are more complex than mini carbs. A potato will take perhaps three hours, mushrooms an hour and a half. Just because something takes longer to digest doesn't mean you can't have it. It means you must learn how to combine it. That is what the Beverly Hills Diet is all about. That is why I call my technique Conscious Combining.

Fats. We don't eat fats by themselves, so we don't need to know how they act alone. We do need to know that they slow down the digestion of whatever it is they are eaten with by as much as several hours or more. But fats don't neutralize any enzymatic action, so you can combine them with a carb or a protein without any serious problem.

Fruit digests the fastest of all. Fruit usually spends, at the most, one hour in your stomach. However, because it is digested so quickly, it combines with *nothing* else. If you eat fruit with any other foods, it will get trapped in your stomach. Think about what happens to a piece of fruit when it's in a hot room for a little while. It ferments.

Remember, all the stomach does to fruit is rot and ripen it and we do not want it to spend any extra time there.

When you miscombine, when you put foods together that are not digested together, you run the risk of two things happening: first, the food will get trapped where it shouldn't and ultimately turn to *fat*; second, because food is not being broken down into nutrients the way it should, you are not getting the nutritional value you need from it. Not only will your hips suffer, but so will your health. Indigestion is far more than gas and heartburn. Indigestion is fat!

Conscious Combining is consciously putting foods together that digest together, foods that work together. By Conscious Combining, not only will you not get fat, you will achieve high health and energy. That's what the Beverly Hills Diet is all about.

Remember:

· Proteins go with other proteins and fats.
· Carbs go with other carbs and fats.
· Fruit goes alone.
· Fats go with either proteins or carbs.

When you mix proteins and carbs, the carbs will usually be trapped in your stomach with the proteins. Your poor stomach can only do one thing at a time, either work or empty. And as long as the protein is there, it has no choice but to work.

If you're fat, you can ill afford so much as a trapped mushroom, a baked potato, or a sprig of parsley! But since man does not live by pasta or steak alone, since the inevitable is that we will miscombine because there are so many marvelous miscombinations—the hamburger with everything on it, spaghetti and meatballs—as well as foods that only exist as miscombinations—those entities unto themselves, the pizza, corned beef on rye, quiche, the "balanced meal"—we *have* to make every "miscombination" count, then know how to correct them. We have to know how to compensate for them. That's coming up a little later. Remember I said you were going to get away with murder, and you will. It's really simple. Staying thin is a product not of what you eat or how much you eat but what foods you eat together and when you eat them. What you eat before them and what you eat after them. By understanding the process, by learning the basics of your body's enzymatic capabilities and taking advantage of this knowledge, you too can obtain slimhood forever. I promise. . . .

THE NEVERS

And I do mean never! I know I told you there were no nevers on my diet. Well there aren't when it comes to food. But who classifies diet soda and artificial sweeteners as food? These seemingly insignificant products can do more to devastate your diet than any other food. I call them the gruesome twosome!

Diet Soda

Sorry. This old diet standby is laden with sodium. (See discussion of salt, p. 42.) But don't despair! Remember, the Beverly Hills Diet lets you eat foods that are important to you—*real* foods. If you were asked to list your ten favorite foods, would diet drinks be on that list? Sodium compounds your bloating problem and thwarts your digestive processes.

Diet drinks are also laden with chemicals such as saccharin. While we're on the subject, you should know that *chemicals* like saccharin totally confound your poor body. Chemicals are a shock to your system, something your body simply was not created to deal with, totally foreign matter, and certainly fully indigestible matter.

Your body is so confused by this foreign matter that, in the process of trying to deal with it, vitamins and minerals are destroyed. Before your body can use food containing chemicals, such as diet soda, it has to detoxify it, draining not only vital nutrients but also energy stores. Think of foods with chemical additives as having to go through a filtering process before their value can be obtained.

Artificial Sweeteners

Don't forget, anything that can't be digested is fattening. Artificial sweeteners can't be digested. They are unnatural chemical compounds that your body simply wasn't built to digest. And, in the process, they foul up the processing of all the foods you eat along with them. Besides, do they really satisfy you?

Interestingly, the only people who don't lose weight on my diet are those who persist with the nevers, those who won't give up their diet soft drinks and their artificial sweeteners.

THE HARDLY EVERS

There are very few hardly evers and they should be put at the bottom of your lists of choices, to be avoided if at all possible and eaten only *rarely*. The truth of the matter is not everyone will have a problem with all or even any of them. You will see for yourself; the scale and your body will tell you. If you gain, if you feel bad after eating them, you should avoid them or eat them with discretion. The choice is yours.

Dairy Products

MILK   First, as we all know, milk of different mammals differs considerably in its composition. What makes us think cows' milk is suited to human needs? How, by the largest stretch of the imagination, do we resemble cows? Why, instead, didn't we fix on goats' milk, dogs' milk, llamas' milk, or pigs' milk? Simple. Because it wasn't as commercially expedient.

Consider further. God created us with the thymus gland, which excretes the enzyme necessary to digest milk. By about four years of age most children begin to lose the use of this enzyme. By puberty, that enzyme is virtually inactive. The thymus gland has shrunk to the size of a pea and is useless.

A key purpose of milk is to promote growth, which is certainly necessary for children. But for adults? It's agreed that one of the reasons Americans are so big is due to our enormous consumption of milk—the growth food.

Interestingly, man is the only mammal who drinks milk after weaning. There are numerous studies indicating that this milk drinking is actually bad for us, that our consumption of dairy products "has life-long serious consequences."* Because most milk is homogenized and pasteurized, the chief ingredient that helps us digest at least the fat content of milk—lecithin—is destroyed by the heating process.

Because we don't really digest milk, we don't obtain the nutrients from it. Obviously, we can't get nutrients from food we can't digest. Touted as nature's most perfect food, even human milk is vastly overrated when compared with other foods, particularly in terms of its protein and calcium content. For instance,

* Frank A. Oske, M.D., and John D. Bell. "Don't Drink Your Milk," *Harper's Bazaar*, 1977.

all whole grains are higher in protein than human milk. Most vegetables are at least twice as high, and bean sprouts and dark-green leafy vegetables are five to eight times as high. Studies show our calcium needs are far below the commercially promoted figure. It could well be that the role of milk in our society is a commercial charade.

Remember that milk is a protein. So that little drop in your morning coffee will make all the carbohydrates that follow it undigestible or fattening.

Probably one of the most difficult things to give up will be the milk in your coffee or tea, especially the coffee you have at the office, since it's usually so terrible. Remember it's just a habit—one you can easily let go of. Try adding some cinnamon for flavor. If yours is one of the offices that has converted from real milk to nondairy creamer, just read the label and that should make it even easier. You really don't want to put all that junk in your body, do you?

CHEESE   It takes ten pounds of milk to make one pound of cheese. Put another way, from one quart of milk you get a small handful of cheese.

If milk is tough, if not impossible, to digest, think what cheese does to your poor stomach without that moisture to ease its course. The harder the cheese, the harder it is to digest. Because it has virtually no moisture, it has to steal moisture from your body. Just like other proteins, only more so. And it suppresses hydrochloric acid, the enzyme necessary to digest fat. So the very enzyme cheese needs more than any other, because of its high fat content, is slowed down.

Another negative: cheese is heavily loaded with salt. If you ever tasted saltless cheese you'd understand why. It's like eating a gum eraser. In addition, most cheeses are loaded with preservatives, stabilizers, and artificial coloring.

Like all other dairy products, cheese creates a great deal of mucus, which coats your lungs and your intestines, making elimination difficult.

Not only does cheese have a lot of salt in it and not only is it in itself as high in calories as any food can be, but cheese also spends more time in your stomach than any other food you eat, it makes anything else you eat after it fattening because anything you eat after the cheese will get trapped in your stomach right along with the cheese. One reason people feel so full after eating cheese is that their stomachs are working so hard they can't deal with anything else. Nothing makes your stomach work harder than cheese and dairy products. Finally as in pasteurizing, processing milk to cheese destroys the lecithin, the ingredient that digests and emulsifies the fat.

YOGURT   Yogurt is a miracle food—a miracle of the marketing place. It's touted as our panacea, the food to make us thin and healthy, the food to make us live forever. This is the food that will cure our ills by killing off bacteria, and, at the same time, cure our ills by creating bacteria. Yogurt has been enshrined among modern-day men.

If milk consumption is on the decline, yogurt's is rocketing, and the dairy industry is happily counting its pennies.

The truth? Yogurt is a low-fat dairy product made by inoculating milk with bacteria. Nothing more. Nothing less. As to its life-lengthening properties, according to well-known Phoenix nutritionist Jeanne Patterson, "There is probably no more correlation of longevity with yogurt than there is to the number of colored telephones within a particular population group."

Nor can man live on yogurt alone—and prosper. By all admissions, yogurt is an incomplete food. Although young rats grow faster when fed yogurt than when fed milk, both products "lack enough iron, Vitamin C, and copper not to sustain life beyond early infancy."* Like milk, yogurt is fairly high in sodium, and salt is not something we want to clog our systems with, as you'll soon see.

The bacteria in yogurt predigest some of the lactose, the natural sugar present in milk products. Some, not all. And if the yogurt is pasteurized, as almost all of it is, this slight advantage is lost because the enzyme and the bacteria are destroyed along with the lecithin that would digest the fat content. Destroy the digesting enzymes and you get zero nutritional value.

We've just been talking about pure, unadulterated yogurt. Add sweeteners or fruit and any possible advantages of raw yogurt are destroyed tenfold.

Remember, cheese and yogurt are also proteins. So adding them to fruits or vegetables will make the carb portion of these foods indigestible. Even one drop will lock all those carbs in your stomach. Hardly worth it, right?

Salt

Salt is a chemical compound consisting of two elements—sodium and chlorine. It's the sodium that causes you all the trouble.

As you know, your body is composed of billions of cells all massed together to create your physical being.

When salt enters your body, it forces water out of your cells and pushes it into the surrounding tissues and gaps between your cells. Because your cells must have water, they call on your body to replace what was taken, and they suck it in from wherever they can get it, putting enormous pressure on the rest of your body.

Your body goes on alert. Water, which would normally be used in other body processes, is now diverted to slake your cells'

* *The New York Times*, August 20, 1980.

thirst. Most of that water will be appropriated from the foods you eat because your cells' needs override all others.

Your body normally passes on most of the water it gets from food to help in the digestion process, especially elimination. It's a constant cleansing process. Water expedites a continual flushing out of your system, ridding it of wastes and potential fat. However, when there is a high concentration of salt in your system, the water thickens and the food and wastes get stuck and can't pass out of your body.

Your body bloats as the liquid accumulates—accumulates in areas where it isn't needed, where it can't be used, where, because of the abnormal demands it places on your organs, it actually works against your system.

You might say so what? It's only water. What difference does that make? Well, a pound is a pound is a pound, whether it's water or whether it's fat. Did you realize that as much as 75 percent of the extra weight you carry around is in a liquid state? Doesn't that make sense when you understand the role water plays in our system and how much of our body weight is water? (See discussion of water, p. 29.)

Also, a high-sodium diet is linked to high blood pressure. Is it any wonder when you look at the pressures it foists on our systems?

Curiously, salt is almost as strong a drug as sugar, because it is such an intense stimulant. Despite its reputation as a flavor enhancer, salt doesn't really make food taste any better. It merely perks up your tongue and assaults your taste buds in a unique way. Once you have been off salt for a while, you will discover a new realm of tastes that had to some extent been masked by the salt.

One reason it's so tough to limit your salt intake is that salt is as pervasive in our food as freckles on a redhead's nose or sand in a desert. Incredibly, only about a third of the salt eaten by the average person is added during cooking or at the table. In its various forms, sodium is used as a curing agent to process food, as a preservative, as a flavor enhancer, and as a leavening agent.

Some foods, like pickles and sauerkraut, are obviously loaded with salt. But did you realize that large amounts of sodium often saturate soups, cheese, canned goods, breads, tuna and most fish, tomato juice, catsup, frozen dinners, even breakfast cereals, ice cream and cake, and, unfortunately, the sacred diet sodas? Some club sodas and some mineral waters are high in salt content, but if you must drink a mineral water, at least choose one with a minimal amount of sodium, such as Evian, Poland Springs, or Perrier. The list, regrettably, is inexhaustible. Food manufacturers are not required to include sodium content on food labels, so even the suspecting sodium-wise eater can be fooled.

If the average person, with ten pounds to lose, gave up salt, within two months he or she would probably lose those ten pounds and never gain them back.

Not everyone is a bloater; not everyone has a salt sensitivity. You will have to discover such things for yourself, learn what's true for you. That is, if you don't already know. When you integrate salt back into your diet, you will experience its effect and then decide whether or not it has a place in your life.

I'm sure you'll find it's worth cutting salt out wherever and whenever you can. After all, don't you want to make every bite count?

Sugar and Other Refined Carbohydrates

In discussing nutrients, I was concerned primarily with their quality, not their quantity. The quality of our output is a direct product of our input. How far would you expect a Rolls-Royce to go on low-grade gasoline? Our health, our energy, our very well-being hinge on the quality of the nutrients our bodies process.

This is especially important with the carbohydrates, which include the ultimate harbinger of bad health—sugar. It is sugar that has saddled carbohydrates with such a bad reputation. Highly refined carbohydrates, such as white flour products, are nearly as bad.

When you eat a piece of candy, the glucose derived from the sugar is not processed in the small intestine. Candy, which contains mostly sugar or sucrose, is converted almost instantly to glucose. This glucose does not have to be processed by your small intestine, but rather it is absorbed by your bloodstream right through the roof of your mouth. It's like getting an instant shot of speed. The effects are much the same. What you feel is a quick high, then a gray low, which triggers a craving for more.

Almost like a narcotic, sugar is clawingly habit-forming. The body will take glucose from wherever it finds it. It doesn't care where it gets it. In some ways it prefers sugar and highly refined starches because the rewards are so instant, so intense—like shooting drugs straight into the bloodstream. Most people on a sugar trip are not getting a usable form of glucose. And because their bodies must have glucose, the cycle intensifies.

Sugar and refined starches really convolute and sap your energy. Most sugar freaks are nervous, high-strung, impatient, and irrational at times. Think about it. How many hyperactive children are hooked on candy, doughnuts, and soft drinks? The sugar demon grabs you by the throat and you can't shake loose. The more your body gets, the more your body craves and the more your body suffers.

Sugar contains no vitamins or minerals. In fact, it creates and inflames a deficiency of the B vitamins which are so vital to your nervous system. Besides devastating the B vitamins in your body, white sugar also causes little pits and the accumulation of mucus in your intestinal wall. The side effect is usually constipation.

Eating should be a process of giving to your body—not taking away from it. Sugar and refined starches take away far more than they give.

THE MEANING OF MAN'S MEDDLING (OR HOW WE TOOK SOMETHING HEALTHFUL AND MADE IT FATTENING)

Food, that wondrous substance that gives up its life to create ours, has inherent within itself all those things that it needs to be digested efficiently in our bodies. Then man came along and started tampering with food to give it more appeal and to make it last longer. Consider:

WHITE BREAD   When man took the grain out of the grain. White bread is supposedly prettier and looks cleaner than brown bread. To achieve this beautiful product, man began with the grain and took out the bran (the fiber and the cellulose) and the germ (the B vitamins), and he then bleached the flour, sapping it of its remaining nutrients.

Eventually, aware of his folly, he did go to the trouble of putting some nutrients back in. Unfortunately, however, nature cannot be duplicated. It is only when foods are in their natural and proper balance that they work for your body, not against it.

ROASTED NUTS   The chief digestive ingredient, lecithin, is roasted right out of the little guys. Heat destroys lecithin.

PASTEURIZED MILK   The pasteurizing zaps the lecithin and thus puts a clamp on any hope we might have had of digesting milk.

OIL   Oils are a vital, natural source of three essential fatty acids your body can only obtain from outside sources. Unfortunately, the common method of extracting oil from its source is through heating (which is how all non-coldpressed oils are processed). The heating destroys those very properties that make oils nutritious, that enable your body to use those fatty acids so critical to its well-being. Once again the lecithin, the key to the oils' digestibility, is destroyed.

HIGH CHOLESTEROL   Most foods are only high in cholesterol because of man's meddling. Anything high in cholesterol is originally high in lecithin as well. Foods are laden with unusable, clotty cholesterol only because its little partner, lecithin, has been destroyed by man's processing. Examples? Butter, milk, and cheese.

To Vitamin or Not to Vitamin?

Your small intestine sits with its little villi at attention eagerly waiting to soak up and disperse all those delectable nutrients your body is processing.

When you take vitamins, they are nutrients in a predigested form, so when they hit the small intestine, it doesn't know what to do with them. Your body's processing job has been appropriated by man, and your small intestine is confused. It is your stomach's action that alerts your small intestine to the fact that nutrients are on the way. If your stomach has no work to do, your small intestine won't know any nutrients are coming. In other words, when predigested nutrients hit your small intestine, it hasn't been alerted, and it must stop and figure out what to do with them.

Each part of the body works in response to another part. So most unfortunately vitamins in pill form are just passed through without being used.

You should know that there are two kinds of vitamins—water soluble and fat soluble.

The Fat-Soluble Vitamins, A, D, E, and K, which are moved through your system by fat, can build up and be stored in your body. Water-soluble vitamins pass right through.

In today's adulterated food world, because so much of our food is overrefined and devoid of vitamins, it is nearly impossible to overdose on vitamins when we obtain them directly from the food we eat, fat-soluble vitamins included.

Vitamin toxicity, or vitamin poisoning, can only happen when you take too many fat-soluble vitamins in pill form.

Although your body will pass all excess water-soluble vitamins through your body, it still has to deal with them. Too many water-soluble vitamins won't cause any harm. But your system still has to divert energy from other sources in deciding what to do about them.

B VITAMINS   There's *always* an exception. Although you are probably getting plenty of vitamins A and C and the other necessary vitamins from your food (or you will be when you combine foods properly), one group of vitamins we can use in supplement form is the B-complex. B vitamins are destroyed by processed food, especially white sugar and flour. Plus, because they are focused primarily in your nervous system, stress and tension deplete them as well.

Thus, the B vitamins are one of the vitamin supplements I recommend you add to your diet, and it will be in the form of nutritional yeast. (See p. 87.)

VITAMIN C   Almost everything you'll be eating on the Beverly Hills Diet is loaded with vitamin C, so you should get more than enough.

THE LOW-CAL EXPOSÉ

Before you begin to apply your new knowledge and experience the joys of the Beverly Hills Diet, I need to vanquish a few much-trumpeted diet myths, because one thing you will have to give up to wear that golden pineapple is any preconceived ideas and opinions you have of what fattening is all about.

Gone are the days of the "diet plate"—the hamburger patty

and cottage cheese. Never again will you have to look a canned peach half in the eye or eat a grapefruit.

When you think of low cal, do you think of foods you crave, or do you imagine bland, slightly off, colorless, limp, plastic-like substances? Low-cal substitutes never really satisfy. They merely intensify and aggravate your food fantasies. If you want heavy, rich ice cream, does flimsy ice milk really take its place? If you lust for thick cream, does the watery, bluish 2-percent-fat milk fulfill your craving?

Diet salad dressings, diet butters, diet mayonnaise, most diet foods, in fact, are glutted with sodium. In almost all "diet" foods, calories are replaced with chemicals, which makes them useless— that is, indigestible. Hence, fattening. At least the calories in food can be turned into energy. Do you want to take a chance on blowing your diet because of an inferior substitute that only increases your love of the real thing?

As far as low-cal plates go, you'll usually find they're not so low-calorie anyway. Let's look at a few of the more prevalent ones.

The Low-Cal Hamburger Plate. Say it's a hamburger patty, a cup of cottage cheese, a canned peach half, and some melba toast. By applying our Conscious Combining knowledge to this appetizing delight, we can see that the canned peach half will ferment in your stomach, and the cottage cheese is loaded with salt and qualifies as cheese, thus holding up the digestion of everything else on the plate. The melba toast turns to alcohol (since it's a grain and fermented grains become alcohol) because it gets stuck in your stomach and along with the peach it ferments.

The Fruit and Cottage Cheese Plate. The cottage cheese traps the fruit in your stomach and causes it to ferment. Instead of getting skinny, you get bloated.

Chef's Salad (also applies to tuna salad, chicken salad, egg

salad, and shrimp salad—all protein based salads). The problem
with these "diet" salads is twofold: they're filled with veggies
that don't get processed properly but instead sit in a lump in your
stomach because of the accompanying protein, and the dressing is
swamped with salt.

Picture the size of your stomach. It's about the size of a small
grapefruit. Yet we're forcing all that bulk to get stuck there. No
wonder your stomach complains!

Grapefruit (and its pal, the orange). I know, *every* diet you
have ever heard of touts the wonders of grapefruit. But, contrary
to public opinion, they have almost no fiber, so they slosh around
in your stomach not doing any particular good. Plus, they have
only a tiny number of active enzymes compared with other, far
more interesting fruits. Eating citrus fruits is like putting a Band-
Aid on a broken leg. They just don't do much. The amount of
vitamin C you derive is wildly overrated. The amount of vitamin A is negligible. And the bulk of those nutrients is concentrated in the seeds, the white membranous lining, and the skin.
When did you last try eating grapefruit skin and orange seeds?

Admittedly, grapefruit is low-cal. But remember, when something is low-calorie it's also low-energy. Put low energy in, and
you get low energy out.

Lemons and Limes. Sad but true, these two are overrated.
What I said about grapefruits and oranges goes for lemons and
limes, too. They contain a special chemical that neutralizes the
all-important pepsin enzyme which digests proteins. Eaten with
or on a protein food—even the smallest squirt on a piece of fish
or chicken—neutralizes the enzyme pepsin and renders the protein indigestible. Which means it's fattening.

Eggs. These are a damned if you do, damned if you don't
item. The ingredient that makes eggs digestible, the lecithin, is
in the yolk and is destroyed when you cook them. On the other
hand, there is an ingredient in the egg white which when eaten

raw destroys B vitamins. The latest craze is to eat only the cooked whites—well, whatever turns you on. I was always a yolk dunker.

Skinless Chicken Breast (and other denuded animal proteins). The skin contains essential nutrients. When you strip it away, you are adversely affecting the digestibility of the fowl. Besides, doesn't it taste better the way nature made it—with the skin on?

Raw Vegetables. Yes, they are low-calorie, but they are low-energy too. So why bother?

Melons. With the important exception of watermelon, which has marvelous enzymatic powers, most melons have no fiber and no digestive enzymes. They are not only hard to digest, but they are bloaters as well.

The Balanced Meal. Frankly, the balanced meal is a sham. If you understand nothing else, appreciate this. Know that the carb portion of that infamous balanced meal is getting stuck in your stomach, that it is not being digested properly because the protein digestion takes precedence. Take meat and potatoes. The potatoes get locked in your stomach and ferment. What are fermented potatoes? Vodka. Why do you think so many people fall asleep after such a meal? Another giveaway? Passing gas, which means the food is fermenting.

The only part of a balanced meal that provides any nutritional value is the protein. Everything else is nullified.

It's the proper balance of carbs, fats, and proteins in our diets that is going to keep us slim, healthy, and energetic. But think about it. Now that you understand the physical laws, isn't the idea of eating them all together as ridiculous as wearing two pairs of shoes at the same time? If the traditional "balanced" meal worked, do you think more than seventy million Americans would be fat?

The enzymatic laws that govern the human body are the

same for everyone. Each individual's capacity to stretch these laws is different. In creating your diet based on my methodology we are going to see just how much *you* can get away with.

THE EMOTIONAL EATER— THE MIND/BODY SPLIT

In developing the Beverly Hills Diet, both for myself and my clients, I have never lost sight of the power of emotions. I know that our hearts are inextricably locked into our eating, that any lifelong diet, by definition, must include not only the mind and the stomach, but our hearts as well.

Those of us who love to eat ("eaters") fall into a special category: almost all of us, at one time or another have been classified as *sensitive*. And it's always said in hushed tones as if sensitivity is a bad thing, something to be ashamed of. Sensitivity is feeling. It's being alive. Eaters are feelers. For us, our need to eat, comes not from a physical hunger but from an emotional hunger.

It's our hearts that need the nourishment, our souls that need to be fed.

We swallow our disappointments, we swallow our hurt, we swallow our anger, we swallow our pride. We eaters, we feelers, will all too often swallow our feelings because publicly and even privately it's the most acceptable way of dealing with them.

We eat when we're excited. We eat when we're sad, when we have too much to do or not enough to do. We eat when we want to escape reality or when we want to connect back to it. When a nightmare wakes us in the middle of the night, food brings reality back into focus.

Eating helps us preserve our sanity. When our pain is intense, eating soothes us—or so we think. It doesn't. It creates a pain all its own. It only prolongs the misery. But we blot this out, obsessed only with the very real, transitory pleasure it affords us.

Eaters are *sensual* people—far more so than noneaters. After all, eating can only be described as a highly sensual experience. While we may not acknowledge this trait of ours, this life energy tends to frighten us. This sensuality is so intense and often so awesome that we often eat not only to satisfy our need but also to mask it, both from ourselves and from others.

Eaters are *high-energy* people, *creative* people, *striving* people. We eat out of frustration, because our power and energy are so scattered and unfocused. If we haven't found our creative avenue, we turn to food. Or we eat to ease off a high, typically after an achievement—after our creativity is spent—to fill the void that comes with accomplishment, the empty space of "what's next?"

Eaters are *wanters*. And we want what we want when we want it, and we want it all *right now*. "More, more, more. . . . Give me more." Too much is never enough. If something is good, more is better. The closest star is never good enough. We've got to have the star farthest away. We're never satisfied. For most of us, if we don't have what we want right now, we think the world will explode. Eaters are not patient people.

We are the masters of setting unrealistic goals. And we are constantly frustrated, constantly wanting.

Because eating is an emotional response to an emotional situation, we get unclear messages from our bodies. Since most of us don't even know where our stomachs are, we can't hear our little cells yelling "Feed me. Nourish *me*. It's my turn." Instead we respond to the heart—only the heart.

As I said earlier, I'm not going to take your heart out of your stomach; I'm going to put your head and your body in. You are going to begin to think about food, really *think* about it.

I'm not going to ask you to give up the one thing that *could* make life work for you.

I'm going to teach you a way of eating that will allow you to be as compulsive as you need to be. I'm not going to make you change an aspect of your personality as inherent as the color of your eyes. I'm not going to make you stop eating, but I am going to make you start *feeling*.

How you feel is based on what you eat. Pure and simple. When I choose not to eat cheesecake, it's not because it doesn't taste good. Are you kidding? It's because it doesn't *feel* good.

Bite by bite, meal by meal, you build your very being, create your very reality. And that reality is based on the quality and the quantity of your energy. Your energy is a magnet; it draws back whatever it puts out. And the bottom line is inescapable: your body, your flesh and blood and energy come from one source— the food you eat.

As you begin to experience the different kinds of energy you get from different foods, you will begin to see how you can control your entire life with food. It is so clear you won't be able to deny it.

Through heightened sensitivity and awareness, by cleansing your body, by getting in touch with yourself, by giving yourself permission to deal with your emotions, by using—not abusing— food, by feeding your body pure, unadulterated food that can easily transform into the nutrients you've been starving for, by living the Beverly Hills Diet, your body will respond. Your *body* will tell you what it *needs*, and you will be able to hear it. Your little skinny voice will begin to talk, and you will listen.

By feeling through cleansing, by taking away all but the most concentrated high-energy foods, you'll be able to abandon that debilitating fat consciousness. You will release your body's skinny voice and let it sing.

Habit will no longer dictate what you eat, nor will eating be only an emotional response to an emotional situation; no longer will hunger be like an assailant coming out of the dark, giving you a quick rabbit punch in the neck. Your heart will say go and your head will say no—and you will begin to listen to your head. You will continue to *love to eat* and *live to eat*, but you will begin to *eat to live*. And as you realize and experience that nothing is leaving the planet, that it will all be here tomorrow and the next day and the day after that for you to enjoy, you get a feeling for later. You begin to think about later and tomorrow and feeling good. So in those moments of madness when all hell breaks loose and you are like a soul possessed and your heart is shouting feed me, feed me; when with wild abandon, without discrimination, you would like to shove it in with both hands, you simply won't be able to. It no longer works; it doesn't feel good.

But you will still eat. The truth is you will always love to eat in those "moments of madness," and that's okay. But you will become aware of a brief moment of clarity in the midst of "being possessed," a moment in which you have a choice. The choice does not have to be *not to eat;* just *not to destroy yourself* in the process. Food will work for you if you'll only let it.

When the need to eat is all-consuming, when your heart is shouting go and your head is shouting no, you will listen to them both. A synergy will develop between your head and your heart, and you will heal your mind/body split. Eating will work for you if you'll only let it.

And you will begin to choose to feel good because it feels a lot better than feeling bad. *Eating* and *feeling good* is what the Beverly Hills Diet is all about.

What have you got to lose?

IV

The
Beverly
Hills
Diet

The TEN COMMANDMENTS—to memorize, internalize, and synthesize into your life to ensure eternal slimhood.

1. Think about food when it doesn't count, so you don't have to think about it when it does.

Make every bite count. Why blow it on things you don't care about or remember? It's not the gourmet dinners that are making you fat. It's the unconscious nibbling . . . on foods that don't count, the foods you'll never miss.

2. If you plan for it, nothing is fattening. (Think about what you want to eat in advance.)

3. What you choose to eat determines what you have to eat.

The diet is your diet, not somebody else's. Build it around the foods you love.

4. Make your scale your best friend and your lover.

It tells you what works and what doesn't work. It doesn't tell you whether you have been good or bad.

5. If you don't have it now, you can have it later. If you don't have it today, you can have it tomorrow. It's not leaving the planet.

That pizza will still be here tomorrow. All the restaurants are not burning down. Nothing is leaving the planet.

6. Think of food in terms of later, for the rest of your life, not for just right *now*.

7. Food is energy—your energy.

How you feel and how the world feels about you depends on your energy. And that energy is a product of one thing—the food you eat. The quality and quantity of your energy is dependent on the food you eat.

8. Make food an experience and experience food. You have permission to enjoy it.

9. Set realistic goals. Don't set yourself up to fail. Don't be a victim.

10. You become a thin person by becoming a thin person, by letting go of the fat person—physically, intellectually, and emotionally.

Confront, acknowledge, and experience the fat person and LET GO. . . .

PHASE ONE:
WEEKS ONE THROUGH THREE

Every fat person is seriously undernourished in some foods and overnourished in others. So in these first few weeks, you will burn, feed, and wash your body to bring it back to its natural nutritional balance. You will burn up your fat by using highly intensive enzymatic fruits, you will feed your body concentrated doses of vitamins and minerals to replace what former eating habits have destroyed, and through washing you will push out the extra water and, once and for all, get rid of the bloating that is an unavoidable adjunct to fat.

If you're overweight you're getting too much of some things and not enough of others. It is the "others" you are about to experience.

Some of these foods you will taste for the first time. For the first week, you will eat a lot of fruit, fresh and organic, if possible. And you can literally eat your heart out—from the time you open your eyes to the time you close them—anytime, anywhere. There is no calorie counting, no food weighing, and unless specified, no portion control. You will not lose more if you eat less. It's *exactly the opposite!*

My diet is designed to maximize your food sensitivity. Thus, you will experience foods in a very specific order—an order designed to help you obtain the ultimate nutrition from the food you eat, and to achieve a healthy, well-balanced, and harmoniously functioning body. Feeling good as well as looking good is what eating is all about.

Do not go hungry. You can and should really get full. You have permission to really eat your fill. Forget about breakfast, lunch, and dinner—eat whenever you are hungry. You will lose weight by feeding your body, not by starving it.

By the third week of the program, when your sensitivity has been adequately developed and your digestive system has been sufficiently rested, you will be able to reexperience the animal proteins: beef, chicken, fish, and eggs, as you desire. Dairy products are the last of the traditional foods to be reintegrated into your diet.

This brief but effective period of food-awareness training will make you think about and experience everything that goes into your body, not in terms of its being an emotional stopgap or a social excuse, but rather in terms of the effect it has on your energy, your state of mind, your state of being. You will begin to think of food not for just right now—but for later, for the rest of your life. You will begin to choose to eat or not to eat something based on how it *feels*. You will become disenchanted with salt and become hooked on pineapples. You will understand that statement, "You are what you eat," and you will feel too good to ever allow yourself to feel bad again. You will find that pot of gold at the end of the rainbow and you will soon be wearing the little golden pineapple, the symbol of eternal slimhood.

You become a thin person by becoming a thin person, by confronting, acknowledging, and letting go of the fat person. By discovering and acknowledging the thin person.

You have to confront and acknowledge what you are now and what you don't want to be before you can become what you want to be.

The nonphysical exercises you do at the end of each week are an imperative part of the process, an integral part of the diet.

Getting thin and staying thin take more than a diet. I cannot stress the nonphysical exercises strongly enough.

For the next five weeks, make a commitment to me and to yourself. Surrender—and just let go! One of the reasons my diet works so well is that you have nothing to think about except getting skinny. You relinquish the responsibility of making choices, eliminating the temptation to cheat. Don't worry, nothing is leaving the planet—it will all still be here tomorrow. All the food you love, or think you love, will still be here whenever you want it.

Important: Any diet, including this one, should be supervised by a doctor. This regimen should *not* be followed by anyone who has diabetes, colitis, hypoglycemia, a spastic colon, ulcers, illeitis, enteritis, diverticulosis, or by anyone who is pregnant or breast feeding.

Rules of the Game— Fixing the Odds in Your Favor

A few urgent and essential final instructions.

1. Weigh yourself every day, and write it all down in the weight section included in the diet. Then tell your weight to someone— the same person—each day. Acknowledge and confront your weight, and let go of it. You confront your weight by weighing yourself. You acknowledge it by writing it down. And you let go of it by telling it to someone. Don't try to remember it. Let it go. If you don't have a scale, buy one immediately. You cannot begin this diet until you do. If you don't weigh yourself, you may not lose weight.

2. Eat the foods only in the order listed. Do not skip around.

Food follows food and one day's program follows another for very specific reasons. Once you have changed foods, don't return to the previous one.

3. If the diet specifies that you should eat a certain amount of a food, eat all that's indicated, even if it means stopping for a while and going back to it. Don't move on to the next food until you do.

4. If an amount is not specified, eat unlimited amounts—as much as you want. Eat until you're full. The more you eat, the more you lose. You are losing weight by feeding your body, not by starving it. Do not let yourself go hungry. Remember, you have permission to really get full.

5. Buy enough, more than you think you'll need. Five pounds of grapes on a grape day is not excessive. Better to freeze leftovers than set yourself up for failure by not having enough.

6. Eat slowly. It isn't how much you eat in how short a time— it's how long you can make the pleasure last.

7. Use frozen food only when fresh food is not available. Do *not* eat canned foods because of the high sodium content.

8. Don't substitute fresh fruit for dried fruit. Dried fruit may be substituted for fresh fruit *only* when fresh or frozen fruits are not available.

9. Eat *only* the foods listed. If something else flies into your mouth, spit it out—quick!

10. Wait two hours between eating *different* kinds of fruits.

11. Wait *three hours* between eating all other kinds of foods— that is, fruit to carb, fruit to protein, carb to carb, carb to protein, protein to protein.

12. All dried fruit must be unsulfured (no sulfur dioxide or preservatives or honey dipped). Soak all dried fruits, except raisins and dates for one hour and then discard the water.

13. All nuts and seeds must be raw and unsalted.

14. Oil must be cold pressed or expeller pressed. (See glossary.)

15. Use unsalted butter only. Use raw butter, if it's available. Raw butter is made from milk that has not been pasteurized or homogenized.

16. Drink water, coffee, and tea only. No diet soda. Noncarbonated mineral waters are preferable to carbonated.

17. No salt, salt substitutes, or powdered seasonings.

18. No artificial sweeteners. Real sweeteners *only* if specified.

19. No nondairy creamer. Milk or cream only if specified.

20. No gum, sugarless or otherwise. Why just chew if you can eat?

21. Fowl must be eaten with the skin. Everything contains essential nutrients.

22. Don't throw anything away. Eat everything, especially the seeds, and eat as many as you can. They are the storehouse of the enzymes, the focus of the nutrients. If you have never tasted grape, papaya, apple, or watermelon seeds, you'll be in for a pleasant surprise.

23. No lime or lemon on anything, *unless* specified. It neutralizes the protein enzyme, pepsin.

24. When alcohol is listed it is optional.

25. The "day" ends when you go to sleep and the new one begins when you wake up—not when the clock strikes midnight. If you wake up in the middle of the night and you will be going back to sleep and you are hungry, continue with the last thing you ate *before* you went to sleep.

Substitutes (Only if You Must)

You should do exactly what's programmed. Each fruit's enzyme has a specific, unique effect, one that cannot be duplicated. In the first few weeks, during the critical burn, feed, and wash stages, the combinations of foods and the order in which they are eaten are particularly important. Remember that the special enzymatic qualities of one fruit can never be exactly duplicated by another.

With these admonitions in mind, and realizing that substitution diminishes the effectiveness of my diet, please resort to the following substitution list *only if absolutely necessary*. After all, who wants to blow it when it really doesn't count?

Substitute Foods List

PROGRAMMED FOODS	SUBSTITUTES
Pineapple	Strawberries
Strawberries	Pineapple
Papaya	Mango, kiwi, persimmon, pineapple, or apples
Prunes	Dried Figs
Bagel	Bread of your choice, prepared without sweeteners.
Almonds	Cashews, sunflower seeds, or brazil nuts
Steak	Lamb, turkey, fish, or veal
Artichokes	Broccoli, asparagus, or brussels sprouts
Chicken	Fish, turkey, or duck

Now that you've thoroughly ingested and digested all the commandments and the rules, you are ready to begin. I emphasize, they were not made to be broken. Following them is vital to your success. They represent the things neither I nor my clients could get away with and still lose weight. And believe me we tried. Down the line you'll be able to stretch some of the rules. I'll let you know where and when. I told you, you only had to give up two things forever and I meant it. There will be a time and a place for everything else. I promise!

Most important, weigh yourself every day, beginning with Day 1. If you don't, my diet will not work for you. The people who do not succeed on my diet are those who either refuse to weigh themselves or insist on slipping in their artificial sweeteners or diet soft drinks. Don't let such foolishness spoil it for you.

Diet for *Week One*

	MORNING	MIDDAY	EVENING
DAY 1 *Weight* ____	Pineapple ——————————————→ 2 Bananas		
DAY 2 *Weight* ____	Papaya ——————————————→ Mango (if available)		
DAY 3 *Weight* ____	Papaya	Pineapple	Papaya
DAY 4 *Weight* ____	Watermelon ————————————————————————→ (if not available, strawberries)		
DAY 5 *Weight* ____	2 Bananas	Dried apricots (8 oz.)	Blueberries
DAY 6 *Weight* ____	Prunes (8 oz.)	Strawberries	2 Bananas
DAY 7 *Weight* ____	Watermelon ————————————————————————→ (if not available, apples)		

PHASE ONE | *Week One*

Week at a Glance:
The Inside Story

During the first week, you will only be having fruit. Don't forget to wait two hours before changing from one fruit to another. Before you decide to make that change, be sure you don't want any more of the first fruit. Once you have finished it, you can't go back to it.

If your day ends with a limited-quantity item, remember that it's the last thing you can eat. Save it until late in the evening so you don't have to go hungry. You might even want to take it to bed with you. Remember, hungry is one thing you'll never be again.

When you buy your pineapple, make sure it is ripe. If it's not it will make your mouth sore. (See Chapter VII on shopping.)

If after looking over the first week's diet, you think you might get tired of pineapple and papaya, don't. Remember, it's their little enzymes that are burning up the fat and digesting all that extra protein that's clogging your system.

Don't think I'd fill your system with pineapple and papaya for no good reason. Pineapples, and to a lesser degree, strawberries, have a high concentration of the enzyme bromaline which interacts with and actuates the hydrochloric acid in your stomach to help burn up the fat.

Papaya, mangoes, kiwis, and persimmons have an enzyme called papain, which interacts with and actuates the pepsin in your stomach to digest all that extra protein and surplus flesh. That's what week one is all about.

Remember the rule: No lemon or lime on your papaya. It will neutralize the very enzyme we are trying to activate.

The Tip Sheet:
Your Daily Bread

On *Day 1*, eat as much pineapple as you want—all day long. You'll probably eat at least two pineapples. Then eat your two bananas. Don't forget the two-hour wait, and don't eat them too early or you'll have nothing left to eat for later. As I mentioned, you might even want to take them to bed with you.

On *Day 2*, six to nine papayas is not excessive.

On *Days 4 and 7*, plan for at least an entire big watermelon. Eat the strawberries on Day 4 and the apples on Day 7 only if you have totally exhausted all possible watermelon sources.

On *Day 5*, if you can't find fresh blueberries, frozen are fine.

Nonphysical Exercise for *Week One:*

The Proud Sheet

Keep a sheet of paper by your bed. Each night, before you go to sleep, write down three things you did that day that you're proud of, things that weren't diet related.

Being fat, whether you are 5 or 105 pounds overweight, is going to bed feeling lousy about yourself. No matter what great things you might have accomplished during the day, the last thing you think about before you go to sleep is the fact that you're still fat.

Stop perpetuating the fat person's consciousness; stop concentrating on your failures.

Accentuate the positive. Let the positive put you to sleep for a change.

Mazeltalk:
The Last Word

Congratulations! Aren't you proud of yourself? You did it! You have lots of energy, you lost weight, and the cleansing process has begun. And you thought you'd never be able to make it through an entire day on watermelon! The best part was that it wasn't even hard.

Now let's talk about the nonphysical exercise. Interesting how differently you felt when you woke up—a little more positive perhaps? Keep the proud sheet going. It's something I still do every night. It really helps me put the day in its proper perspective.

How many pounds did you say you lost? Go ahead! *Brag about it!*

Now you are ready for week two.

Diet for *Week Two*

	MORNING	MIDDAY	EVENING
DAY 8 *Weight* _____	Prunes (8 oz.)	Strawberries	Raisins (8 oz.)
DAY 9 *Weight* _____	Grapes ——————————————————————→		
DAY 10 *Weight* _____	Grapes ——————————————————————→		
DAY 11 *Weight* _____	3½ Bagels or 8 oz. of your favorite bread (unsweetened)	(2 Tbs. unsalted butter for day) ——————→	3 ears of corn on the cob
DAY 12 *Weight* _____	Pineapple ——————————————→		Mazel Salad with Mazel Dressing (*see* menus and recipes)
DAY 13 *Weight* _____	Apples ——————————————————→		Baked potatoes with 2 Tbs. butter

	MORNING	MIDDAY	EVENING
DAY 14 *Weight* _____	Mango (if not available, papaya) ——————————————→		

PHASE ONE | *Week Two*

Week at a Glance:
The Inside Story

Don't forget that the purpose of these first few weeks is to cleanse your body, to get it ready for Conscious Combining. We do this through the three-part enzymatic process of burning, feeding, and washing.

Last week, we focused primarily on the burning process, although we did feed and wash your system as well. Although we will continue burning and washing in week two, we will concentrate on the feeding phase.

It is the concentration of minerals in the dried fruits and the grapes that will help correct an imbalance in your body's mineral content. This imbalance is generally caused by the traditional American diet, a diet high in chemicals, sugar, and processed food. A diet that provokes a strong mineral imbalance as well as clogging your system.

Unfortunately, most commercially dried fruits are processed with sulfur dioxide. If we start putting chemicals back into our system with these fruits, we're defeating our purpose. Be sure to buy your dried fruits at a health-food store or else make sure they are not touched by chemicals. "No sulfur dioxide added" will be on the package.

Keep in mind the rule that all dried fruits, except raisins, must be soaked in water to replenish their moisture—a corrective for man's meddling.

One of the reasons fruit is 80 percent water is that the water helps in its digestion. When the water is removed, the dried fruit is difficult to digest, and a bit too highly concentrated for your body to take advantage of it.

The enzymes in the grapes, another primary feed fruit, will interact with the enzymes in your large intestine to help clean it out. It's going to have a Roto-Rooter effect as it cleanses your intestinal wall.

If sugar has been a regular part of your diet, grapes will also help pry your fat loose by pushing stored sugar residues out of your body. Even if you are not a sugar-holic, you need the grapes because so much of the food you eat has hidden sugar in it— catsup, salad dressing, toothpaste, mouthwash, salt, powdered seasonings. The list goes on and on. . . . You get the idea.

The Tip Sheet:
Your Daily Bread

Now that other foods have been reintegrated into your diet, don't forget the rule requiring *a three-hour wait between any foods other than from one fruit to another fruit. Remember fruit to fruit is two hours; fruit to anything else is three hours* (that is, fruit to carb, fruit to protein, also carb to protein, protein to protein). The waiting time is vital. I don't mean 1 hour and 50 minutes or 2 hours and 20 minutes.

On *Day 8,* you have two limited-quantity items. Pace yourself. Eat all your prunes before eating your strawberries. When I specify eight ounces, I mean eight ounces, no more, no less. Even if you stop and start with those prunes, which, by the way, lots of Beverly Hills' dieters do, eat the full eight ounces. Then you may begin your strawberries. Remember you have a limited quantity of raisins and they are the last thing you will be eating today so don't stop your strawberries or start those raisins too early, or you'll be sorry. Pace yourself.

Days 9 and 10, grapes are great for compulsive eaters. You can just keep popping them in. Most people eat about five pounds a day. Mix the colors, eat the seeds. Have fun and eat as much as you want.

On *Days 11 and 12,* you'll have to pace yourself again. On

Day 11, eat your bread during the day and your corn-on-the-cob at night. Don't eat all your bread in the morning or you'll get hungry in the afternoon. Don't worry, you'll have enough.

Believe me, these quantities have been tested on very big eaters. They did not experience hunger and neither will you.

Corn, by the way, is a good intestinal sweep—like a little broom. If you put too much butter on it, though, it will stick instead of sweep.

Day 12 means pineapple all day. Save your salad for the evening. The best way to eat salad is in one sitting but you can "nosh" if you want. Be sure to chew it well.

On Day 13, you can eat any and all kinds of apples. Don't forget, eat the seeds and the skin. Try to find unwaxed apples.

There's no limit to how many potatoes you can eat. The average Beverly Hills dieter usually eats two big ones. If you really want another, eat a third. But keep in mind that potatoes swell in your stomach, and if you eat too much, you will feel uncomfortable. Believe me, I know. Potatoes are like thirsty sponges. They'll soak up as much butter as you give them. Don't use more than two tablespoons.

Day 14. If you're lucky and that rare fruit, the magical mango, is available to you, count on eating at least five of them. If mangoes are not to be had, eat papaya. The result will be the same.

Nonphysical Exercise for *Week Two*:
The Three Questions

Get ready for all the positive feelings your new body is about to bring your way. Ask three very important people in your life the three things they like best about you. Don't comment on their responses. Just listen, *really* listen. Go home and write them down. Revel in the positive information, and know that this is just the beginning of what is going to become a steady stream of compliments. You might want to use this space to write the compliments; that way you will have some ready support when you need it.

Mazeltalk:
The Final Word

Look at that! Not only did you lose weight, but you did it eating corn-on-the-cob and baked potatoes! And you weren't hungry, were you? Not only that, you still haven't thought about cheating. Well, maybe once, for a minute and a half.

Interesting isn't it, what people think of you. Are you surprised?

You are weighing yourself and telling your weight to someone every day, aren't you?

Well onward and downward. Let's see what week three has in store.

Diet for *Week Three*

	MORNING	MIDDAY	EVENING
DAY 15 *Weight* _____	2 Bananas	Raisins (8 oz.)	Almonds (4 oz.) *or* cashews, (4 oz.)
DAY 16 *Weight* _____	Pineapple ————————————➤		L.T.O. with Mazel Dressing (see recipes)
DAY 17 *Weight* _____	Zucchini	String beans and mushrooms ◄———2 Tbs. Butter———➤ for the day	Artichokes *or* broccoli and cauliflower
DAY 18 *Weight* _____	Kiwi (if not————————————————➤ available, papaya)		Papaya
DAY 19 *Weight* _____	Apples◄————————————➤		Steak *or* lobster with unsalted butter

	MORNING	MIDDAY	EVENING
DAY 20 *Weight* _____	Chicken ————————————————→		
DAY 21 *Weight* _____	Watermelon ————————————→ (if not available, pineapple)		

PHASE ONE | *Week Three*

Week at a Glance:
The Inside Story

The main goal of the Beverly Hills Diet in the third week is still to lose weight. While we are still burning, feeding, and washing, we will also be reintegrating some of those more familiar foods. Like the proteins. First we're adding nuts, a special kind of protein, and later in the week, you will have your choice of steak or lobster—as much as you want. And then chicken—skin and all —cooked any way you like it best. This week you begin having choices. Make up your mind before the week begins, fill in the blanks, and that's it. Once you have made your decision, do not change it. Remember it's only food. If you choose cashews this time, next time you'll have almonds.

The Tip Sheet:
Your Daily Bread

On *Day 15*, don't forget to wait three hours between your raisins and nuts, which must be unsalted and raw. Eat all 8 ounces of your raisins, please.

On *Day 17*, remember, no salt, no salt substitutes, and no powdered seasonings on your veggies. You can have two tablespoons of unsalted butter for the day and you can use as much Mazel Dressing as you like. You are eating zucchini and string beans to balance the acidity and alkalinity of your system—your pH.

On *Day 19*, have your last bite of apple at least three hours before your steak or lobster. Use some discretion as to how much unsalted butter you use. Fresh garlic or pepper only on the steak.

Day 20 is chicken day. That means chicken cooked any way you want it, but, remember, no salt, salt substitutes, or powdered seasonings. You can, however, use fresh herbs. And you can sauté or fry it in a moderate amount of cold-pressed oil or unsalted butter. Use your imagination. This is a fun day. And eat the skin.

Don't buy chicken that's already prepared since it's probably preseasoned with all of the above. The same for fried-chicken carryouts.

On *Day 21*, if you absolutely cannot find watermelon, substitute with pineapple only.

Nonphysical Exercise for *Week Three*:
Seeing Yourself As Others See You

Sorry, you don't. Do you think anyone else focuses on your cellulite? You have devoted your existence to your imperfections. We know where all our negative parts are. But we never see the wonderful side of ourselves. We refuse to acknowledge our new bodies. I want you to start examining your beautiful new body and watch it emerge. If you don't own a full-length mirror, now is the time to get one. You cannot do the exercises without it, and the exercise is integral to your weight loss.

Spend ten minutes, nude, in front of your full-length mirror looking at yourself. What's the best part of you. Where are you getting thinner? Write it down, or, better yet, brag to someone about it. Is a bridge built before it is someone's idea? Well how do you expect to create a fabulous body if you don't see it.

The hardest part of this experience is ignoring the parts you always chose to see in the past—THE FAT. As soon as you catch yourself back there again, focusing on your fat, just force your attention away. Soon it will be easy to focus on those emerging hip bones and slimmer thighs, and before you know it, there won't be any bad parts left.

84

Mazeltalk:
The Final Word

Congratulations! You made it through basic training. When did you ever never cheat before? What power; what control; you're terrific! If you only had ten pounds to lose, you've undoubtedly lost it by now. Aren't you feeling wonderful? Did you ever imagine that a diet that *works* could be so much fun? So easy?

If you reach your weight goal at the end of these three weeks, go directly onto the maintenance program. If you reach your goal before the end of the three weeks, it is vital that you still complete this phase of the diet to thoroughly cleanse and effectively burn, wash, and feed your body and thus prepare it for maintenance.

If you lose too much, you can always gain it back.

PHASE TWO:
WEEKS FOUR AND FIVE

DISCOVERING THE POT OF GOLD

Most of you will not have lost all your extra weight yet. Many of you still have a long way to go. Whatever the case, you are on your way, and you will reach your goal. You can be sure of this. The diet gets better and better, and you are getting stronger and stronger and thinner and thinner. So relax and enjoy yourself as we move along and go all the way to the end of the rainbow where your pot of gold waits—"eternal slimhood."

Now that your body has been burned, fed, and washed, the proper nutritional balance has been restored. Now, it is time to create a truly balanced diet, to introduce the proper harmony between food groups and nutrients. Remember, if you're overweight you're getting too much of something and not enough of something else. We don't want to perpetuate that condition.

Fruits will continue to play a starring role because the burning, feeding, and washing must continue. Animal protein on a regular basis and combined meals will be introduced now—a proper balance both physically and psychologically. I, especially, know that man does not live by pineapple alone.

Supplements

Important: In Phase Two, it is vital that the following supplements be included in your daily diet:

On arising in the morning, eat two tablespoons of unprocessed bran flakes, and then drink a hot beverage. Wait forty-five minutes before eating anything else.

Bran is the ultimate nutritional broom. It is important that you eat this high-fiber food only on an empty stomach so it doesn't get trapped behind other foods and bloat your stomach. It is virtually impossible to overload your body with fiber.

At 4:00 p.m., eat one tablespoon of nutritional-yeast flakes in a small amount of water. I make mine the consistency of peanut butter. Do not eat for one hour before or after taking the yeast. The reason for the hour's wait is that, like all other foods, the yeast can get trapped in your stomach instead of being properly and efficiently digested.

Remember, you're taking the yeast to keep your body's vitamins in balance. Even if your diet doesn't include foods that deplete the B complex vitamins, which is highly unlikely, a stressful life-style will still sap your store of these vital nutrients.

At bedtime, eat two tablespoons of unhulled, raw sesame seeds. Sesame seeds are the richest source of calcium on the planet. They also provide your body with the three essential fatty acids that you can only get from foods. Sesame seeds—this wonderful, munchy, bedtime snack—will also supply your body with additional fiber. An added bonus is that their concentrated calcium helps you sleep by relaxing your nervous system.

Combined Meals

As I told you, man does not live by pineapple alone, or by potato alone. If that were the case, how could I ever expect you to think of this as a way of life? Enter the "combined meal."

What exactly are the combined meals I keep talking about? So far you have experienced only one type of meal—the Mono Meal, one thing at a time, either one protein, one fruit, or one carb.

Before I knew about the physical laws that govern the human body, I had already begun to limit my combinations. I knew that as long as there were many combinations of tastes available to me, my mouth would keep on going. The tendency is to overeat when you have a lot of choices at any one time. Think about buffets, cocktail parties, and multicourse sit-down meals. Keep this tendency in mind as you return to combined meals. Remember that the mouth of an eater is like the keys of a finely tuned piano—each bite rings out a different note, and we are only happy when they are all playing in harmony. The tunes are endless.

The number of combined meals you can safely get away with really has to do with your ability to know when enough is enough. It is imperative that you exercise control when you eat combinations. Don't let your heart take over. Eat like a human being, not a fat person.

The following combinations refer to *specific meals* or *individual eating experiences, not entire days.*

OPEN FRUIT Fruit, combined with wine, champagne, or brandy. One fruit only. Fruits do not combine with one another, as you'll discover when you begin your own experimenting. Examples:

· Strawberries and champagne
· Grapes and wine

OPEN CARB The combination of three carbs, with not more than two being maxi carbs. Remember, the maxi carbs are bread, potatoes, pasta, grains, artichokes, alcohol, and most desserts. (*See* Chapter III *for an inclusive list.*) Also, keep in mind that fats go with anything. Examples:

· Stir-fried vegetables, sake, and rice
· The Bjorg Special: salad, bread and butter, and chocolate cake
· Artichoke, baked potato, and steamed asparagus

OPEN PROTEIN The combination of any three proteins from any category, excluding nuts. Nuts combine only with other nuts. Examples:

· Clams, oysters, and lobster
· Mixed grill: lamb chop, veal chop, and a fillet of beef
· Cracked crab, steak, and cheesecake
· Chicken-liver omelette and bacon

OPEN MISCOMBINATION   There are two types:

1. *One carb and one protein.* You follow the rule of eating the protein last. Eat the carb first, and once you have taken your first bite of protein, do not go back to the carb. Examples:

- Salad and steak
- Asparagus and fillet of sole
- Chocolate cake and chicken. (Yes, here dessert will precede the chicken.)

2. *The entity unto itself.* Since we can only get away with just so many miscombinations this is the type of open miscombination you'll probably most often choose, the type that really feeds your heart and your soul. Frankly, was the asparagus or the salad worth it? Examples:

- Hamburger with everything on it
- Quiche
- Canneloni
- Spaghetti and meatballs
- Club sandwich
- Linguini with clam sauce
- Tuna-salad sandwich
- Corned beef on rye
- Pizza

How far can *you* stretch the rules? Each individual is different. The bottom line is that the carb in the miscombination won't digest properly. This does not mean you can't ever have those things you really love, but, rather, that you will carefully choose the occasions and make them count.

Because a miscombination always includes protein, any meal that follows it on the same day *must* be a protein meal—preferably a Mono Protein. If you had a miscombination at breakfast, it's protein for the rest of the day.

OPEN DESSERT That means dessert instead of a meal. If it is in lieu of a midday meal, choose two normal human portions. If it is in the evening, choose three normal human portions.

If it's ice cream at night, allow yourself one and one half pints maximum. Open Dessert means just that—any dessert from chocolate chip cookies to a lemon soufflé, from cherries jubilee to a raspberry custard tart.

If it isn't the last meal of the day, it should be followed by a protein meal.

RESNICK OPEN This one's named after a drinking client. Some of us can't eat and drink at the same time without gaining weight, so we have to make a choice. If that choice is to drink, then it is a Resnick Open.

Just like eating, a Resnick Open should be separated from other foods by two or three hours. If you go on Resnick Open and you are going to wine, you must do so after fruit, and it's a two-hour wait. If it's fruit to a grain alcohol, it's three hours.

You can only drink wine or champagne on a fruit day. If you had a carb lunch, you can't drink anything other than a grain alcohol. If you ate protein, you can't drink at all.

Remember, once you are off fruit, you can't go back to it. Wine is fruit. Alcohol is carb. Once you have eaten protein, you can't eat or drink anything other than protein. I don't know of any alcohol made from cow's blood.

OPEN HUMAN At long last, the category you've all been waiting for, the one that proves your little skinny voice has been set free and that you can indeed eat with some sort of discipline.

Open Human means eating anything and everything in any

order you wish. Combining all foods but doing it with discipline. Just because something is good, that doesn't mean more is better. The idea of Open Human is not to pig out and gain weight but to eat like a "mensch" (see Glossary) with one hand, one bite at a time, enjoying and experiencing each bite.

One of the big problems on an Open Human is knowing when enough is enough. On an Open Human, follow the lead of a skinny person—not an anorexic skinny person who you know will either go home and vomit or starve themselves for a week—but an authentic skinny person, a person who knows when he or she has had enough to eat, no matter how grand the food. Remembering all the while that if you don't eat it all now, there will be some left for tomorrow, and if you don't have it tomorrow, maybe again next week. It will all be here. Nothing is leaving the planet. If you successfully make it through your Open Human, if you don't gain weight, one thing will leave the planet —your fear of never being able to eat like a real human being.

On an Open Human, you should follow that skinny person's lead. Ideally, you will be able to identify a thin individual and match him or her bite for bite. While you might not find yourself totally satisfied, you probably won't go hungry either.

At a glorious dinner party, I watched Herb Rousso eat two bites of spinach florentine and stop. Although I could easily have consumed the entire dish, as an experiment I followed his example. When he left most of his tender, glistening manicotti, so did I, and there were tears in my eyes when the waiter swept mine away. Yet, it worked. I survived without gaining so much as an ounce, eating like a "normal" human through all twelve courses of that fabulous meal: tasting, enjoying, and experiencing each morsel that crossed my lips.

Most enjoyable of all? There was no cloying guilt, no upset stomach, no miserable recriminations, and no extra pounds the next day on the scale. And when I thought about it—no hunger;

I really was full when we finished. Also, I knew that if I had managed to eat that wonderful meal with moderation and thus without gaining weight, I could do it all over again tomorrow and the next day and the next. If I had made it the last supper, that is exactly what it would have become. I didn't and it didn't.

Remember, it's not how much you can eat in how short a time; it's how long you can make the pleasure last. So eat and enjoy. And prove you have a skinny heart.

Your best bet for weight loss is the Mono Meal. Second best weight-losing choice is Open Carb or Open Protein. Needless to say, Open Human or Open Miscombination meals are no guarantee that you will lose or even maintain. That's up to you.

And now it's time for week four.

Diet for *Week Four*

	MORNING	MIDDAY	EVENING
DAY 22 *Weight* ____	Papaya or kiwi	Hamburger with everything on it *or* tuna-salad sandwich	Fish
DAY 23 *Weight* ____	Pineapple ⟶		2 glasses wine *or* champagne
DAY 24 *Weight* ____	1½ Breads	Mini Mazel Salad	Stir-fried vegetables, rice, and sake *or* your choice of any Open Carb meal
DAY 25 *Weight* ____	Apples ⟶		Popcorn
DAY 26 *Weight* ____	Prunes (8 oz.)	Raspberries or strawberries	Pasta with bread and butter *or* with 2 vodkas

	MORNING	MIDDAY	EVENING
DAY 27 *Weight* _____	Grapes ——————————————————————→		
DAY 28 *Weight* _____	Cherries (if ————————————→ not available, strawberries)——————————→		Raisins (8 oz.)

PHASE TWO | *Week Four*

Week at a Glance:
The Inside Story

Now the fun really begins. Don't be scared. You really will lose weight on popcorn and hamburgers with everything on them.

This week you will have to wait a bit between different foods —at least three hours. So pace yourself. And be aware!

You should continue to soak your dried fruit. The alcohol is optional.

The Tip Sheet:
Your Daily Bread

On *Day* 22, your first miscombination, note that's a hamburger, not a cheeseburger. You can have *anything* else on it that makes it a hamburger for you—mustard, ketchup, and mayo—but forget the chile unless it's really essential. And please, pass on the pickle since it has too much salt.

On *Day* 23, if you choose to have wine or champagne, you can continue to munch on your pineapple straight through the evening—an Open Fruit—or you can separate them and do a Resnick Open (See Page 91.)

On *Day* 24, one serving of bread equals two bagels, two croissants, or two slices of bread. (See pages 184 and 197 for the recipes for Mini Mazel Salad and the Chinese Stir-Fry Vegetables.)

On *Day* 25, no salt or butter on your popcorn. No butter because it thwarts the popcorn's work as an intestinal broom. Count on about one cup of unpopped popcorn. Pop it in cold-pressed corn oil.

Yes, indeed, *Day* 26 is pasta with pleasure. Remember, not so much as a whisper of cheese or meat. It's the presence of protein that makes pasta so fattening. Trust me. Try your pasta with butter or oil, a little fresh parsley, and garlic—Pesto Mazel—and you're in heaven. For further inspiration, look over my pasta recipes. Note that in addition to the pasta, you can have bread and butter *or* two servings of vodka—an Open Carb meal.

On *Day 28*, try to find cherries. They feed, they cleanse, and they do wonderful things for your joints by breaking up deposits. If you find them, eat them all day. Otherwise, you will have to go with the strawberry/raisin combo.

Nonphysical Exercise for *Week Four*:
The Sharon Assignment

"I hate to be fat!"
"I don't have to be fat anymore!"
"I'll never be fat again!"

Can you imagine saying that to anyone, let alone a stranger? Remember, you have to acknowledge and confront your weight before you can let go of it. You have carried it around long enough. Go up to three people—friends, or preferably strangers —and repeat the above with conviction. No preliminaries or explanations. Write down how it makes you feel.

Sharon was at a plateau, that inevitable period when you stop losing weight (see page 132), when I devised this little game for her to play. The day after she did this in an elevator full of strangers, she not only broke her plateau, but she also lost 3½ pounds. Try it. It's fun.

Mazeltalk:
The Final Word

Now, do you believe it? Do you have any excuses left? You ate pasta and hamburger and popcorn, and you still lost weight!

One by one, every excuse you had for blowing it is being taken away. . . . One by one, every excuse you had for being fat is being taken away. . . . Soon you will have the body you've always dreamed of. You are about to experience your dream come true. I'm not going to leave you with one excuse. You've come this far—you have a skinny potential; your perseverance has proved it.

Diet for *Week Five*

	MORNING	MIDDAY	EVENING
DAY 29 *Weight* _____	Grapes ————————————————→		2 glasses wine or champagne
DAY 30 *Weight* _____	Figs, fresh or dried	Dates (6 oz.)	Potatoes, any style with Mazel *or* L.T.O. Salad, (see recipes, Chapter VI) and vodka *or* Open Dessert
DAY 31 *Weight* _____	Mango (if not available, papaya)		Pineapple →
DAY 32 *Weight* _____	Eggs and toast	Mono Protein	Open Protein
DAY 33 *Weight* _____	Kiwi (if not available, papaya) ————————————→		Papaya

	MORNING	MIDDAY	EVENING
DAY 34 *Weight* _____	Pineapple————————————————➤		Mazel Salad and vodka
DAY 35 *Weight* _____	Watermelon————————————————➤ or grapes		

PHASE TWO | *Week Five*

Week at a Glance:
The Inside Story

Inch by inch, pound by pound, slimhood is becoming a reality. I know. You didn't lose twenty pounds last week. But there you go with your unrealistic expectations again. Stop disavowing each pound you've lost as unimportant. Accept the place you are today, and feel your body as it is today. You've come a long way in a single month!

Remember, you become a thin person by becoming a thin person, by confronting, acknowledging, and letting go of the fat person.

So relax, let go, and have fun. You'll only have to get skinny once.

Onward and downward!

In week five, we're going to stabilize the burn, feed, and wash cycle, by applying all three processes simultaneously. We're also going to continue to reintegrate all those foods that make life worth living.

You'll notice that this week there is only one food with a limit on quantity. That's because I hope you are learning when enough is enough, experiencing that just because something is good, more is *not* better.

Of course, you are still weighing yourself each and every day, aren't you? As well as writing it down and telling it to the same person? It's even more important as your diet becomes more discretionary, more liberating. Unless you are weighing yourself, you won't know what's working and what's not.

And, of course, you're doing the nonphysical exercise that follows each week's diet. Remember, my Beverly Hills Diet feeds all of you, not just your physical form. If slimhood is to become a reality for your mind as well as your body, your soul as well as your stomach, the nonphysical exercises are essential.

Keep your proud sheet going; don't stop looking in the mirror; keep playing the Sharon Assignment. Ask more than three people the questions. Use the exercises to discover your skinny self.

The Tip Sheet:
Your Daily Bread

On *Day 29*, remember that the wine or champagne is optional. This can be either an Open Fruit or a Resnick Open.

Try to get fresh figs on *Day 30*. Yes, it does say dessert! This evening choose between potatoes, a Mazel *or* L.T.O. Salad, and vodka, *or* an Open Dessert—any combination of three dessert servings of your heart's desire. By potatoes any-style, I mean French fries, chips (unsalted are available at health-food stores), hashbrowns, or even eggless latkes, also known as potato pancakes. (See recipes, page 189.) You name it, as long as it isn't contaminated with so much as a smidgen of protein or a dash of salt. Yes, you can have two tablespoons of butter.

On *Day 32*, we bring back that old friend, the traditional breakfast. Prepare your eggs just as you would have before I entered your life. You can even butter your toast, as long as it's unsalted butter.

Don't forget the rule that once you've eaten protein, you must stick with protein for the rest of the day. If you never break this one rule, the protein rule, I promise you will never get fat. It's so firmly embedded in my soul that I would no more break it than commit murder. That's why Day 32 follows through with protein. Remember, Mono Protein means a single protein, while

Open Protein means you can combine a number of different proteins.

On *Day 35*, try to find some watermelon before you turn to grapes.

Nonphysical Exercise for *Week Five*:
Positive Talkback

By now you're hooked—you have become a Conscious Combiner. The only problem is that the rest of the world doesn't understand the world of our little golden pineapple. Those questions! "Are you still on that crazy diet?" "When are you going to eat like a normal person?" "Isn't it boring?" "Isn't the Beverly Hills Diet unhealthy?" "When are you getting off it?" And best of all, "You're getting too thin!"

Respond to each question in Positive Talkback as follows:

"Funny, you should mention that. I'm the skinniest person here!" (It would be wise to assess the crowd first.)

"Do you think it's easy being gorgeous?" (My favorite.)

"Isn't it boring being fat? (With a straight face.)

"Why would I stop doing something that makes me feel so good?"

"Thank you!"

Mazeltalk:
The Final Word

See? You'll never have to blow your diet again. If you plan for it, nothing is fattening. Isn't it fun learning to make every bite count—and getting thin at the same time?

You can stay on Phase Two for as long as you have weight to lose. Once your body is burned, fed, and washed, these two weeks will promote a most efficient weight loss.

All of us, after all, are human. So if you have a compulsion to blow it without blowing it, if you need to take a week off, move on to Week Six. It's okay; you don't *have* to lose weight every second. Life doesn't have to be all losing or gaining—what about just *being*? You have permission to blow it. Blow it, that is, without blowing it.

PHASE THREE | *Week Six*

EATING TO YOUR HEART'S CONTENT WITHOUT EATING YOUR HEART OUT . . .

OK, OK! You've had it with diets and dieting. You want a week off. You need a Mexican-food fix, a pizza, just a "regular" meal! Blowing It Without Blowing It is giving yourself permission to eat. But, *please*, eat like a normal person, with one hand, one bite at a time. Just because something is good doesn't mean that more is better. If you don't eat it all today, it will still be here tomorrow.

Each bite you take is a commitment. It's *your* diet, even when you're blowing it, because what you choose to eat determines what you have to eat. You can give yourself permission to blow it because you are making a commitment to making it work, eating what you have to eat *next* to make it work. Now, you'll learn how to make even the most fattening food nonfattening. So, Blow It Without Blowing It. Give yourself permission but, if you make it the Last Supper, it will be.

If you eat as if there is no tomorrow, there won't be. That fat consciousness, that thing that forces us to cram all of it in right now, comes from not being able to have it tomorrow because we think it's fattening. It's only our attitude and our actions that make it fattening.

If you make a pig out of yourself, you'll become one. Pigs stuff themselves until they can barely move—is it really still necessary for you to do that?

Caution: Do not go to Week Six until you have completed all five weeks of Phase One and Phase Two of the Beverly Hills Diet.

Diet for *Week Six*

	MORNING	MIDDAY	EVENING
DAY 36 *Weight* _____	Papaya ————————————————►		Pizza, as you like it, *or* Mexican dinner
DAY 37 *Weight* _____	Pineapple ————————————————►		Strawberries
DAY 38 *Weight* _____	Watermelon ————————————————————————————►		
	(if not available, grapes)		
DAY 39 *Weight* _____	Papaya or kiwi ————————————►		Chinese, Japanese, *or* Middle Eastern ethnic dinner (Mexican and Italian *excluded*)

	MORNING	MIDDAY	EVENING
DAY 40 *Weight* _____	Watermelon —————————————————————————▶ (if not available, strawberries)		
DAY 41 *Weight* _____	Papaya —————————————————▶		Traditional "balanced" American dinner
DAY 42 *Weight* _____	Pineapple, papaya, mango, ——————————————▶ strawberries, or kiwi		Popcorn (no salt or butter)

PHASE THREE | *Week Six*

Week at a Glance:
The Inside Story

Don't be alarmed if your weight fluctuates from one day to the next. What goes up must come down. It's the law of gravity, and all those little enzymes are going to prove that law for you.

All of the notoriously fattening foods that have been included in this Blowing-It week are only fattening because they are hard to digest. Now you're really going to see the enzymes in action—burning, feeding, and washing. You saw how the enzymes made you lose weight. Well the same enzymes are going to help you maintain your weight, no matter what they come up against. Now you'll really become a believer.

If you follow this week's program exactly, and I underline *exactly;* if you don't stuff yourself until you are like a beached whale unable to move away from the table; if you eat like a mensch, with one hand, one bite at a time, always being aware of tomorrow, then you will weigh the same at the end of the week as you did at the beginning.

On Week Six of the Beverly Hills Diet, we're really flouting all the rules. You will hopefully experience that salt is really an assault, that cheese is not as wonderful as you thought it was, and that your Mexican meal was no great shakes!

Mazeltalk:
The Final Word

You see? It worked, didn't it? Those enzymes really work! In your wildest dreams, did you ever imagine you could eat the way you did this week—and not gain a single pound?

After completing Week Six, to continue losing you have two options: Go back to Week Two, and follow through Phase Two for the quickest possible weight loss; or, you can simply repeat Weeks Four and Five indefinitely. While the weight loss will be slightly slower, psychologically it will be easier to stick with because you'll have more choices. Go back to Week One only if you have really gorged for more than a month. To optimize weight loss, don't go on Week Six more often than every six weeks.

If maintenance is now your goal, move on to the program outlined in Chapter VI. Congratulations, skinny! You proved me right again, and *I'm proud of you.*

The Beverly Hills Diet: A Synopsis

	MORNING	MIDDAY	EVENING
Week One			
DAY 1	Pineapple		2 Bananas
DAY 2	Papaya		Mango, if available
DAY 3	Papaya	Pineapple	Papaya
DAY 4	Watermelon (if not available, strawberries)		
DAY 5	2 Bananas	Dried apricots (8 oz.)	Blueberries
DAY 6	Prunes (8 oz.)	Strawberries	2 Bananas
DAY 7	Watermelon (if not available, apples)		
Week Two			
DAY 8	Prunes (8 oz.)	Strawberries	Raisins (8 oz.)
DAY 9	Grapes		
DAY 10	Grapes		
DAY 11	3½ Bagels or 8 oz. of your	(2 Tbs. unsalted	3 ears corn on the cob

116

	MORNING	MIDDAY	EVENING
	favorite bread (unsweetened)	butter for the day)	
DAY 12	Pineapple		Mazel Salad with Mazel Dressing (see menus and recipes)
DAY 13	Apples		Baked potatoes (2 Tbs. butter
DAY 14	Mango (if not available, papaya)		Papaya

Week Three

	MORNING	MIDDAY	EVENING
DAY 15	2 Bananas	Raisins (8 oz.)	Almonds (4 oz.) or cashews (4 oz.)
DAY 16	Pineapple		L.T.O. with Mazel Dressing (see recipes)
DAY 17	Zucchini	String beans and mushrooms (2 Tbs. butter for the day)	Artichokes *or* broccoli and cauliflower

	MORNING	MIDDAY	EVENING
DAY 18	Kiwi (if not available, papaya)		Papaya
DAY 19	Apples		Steak *or* lobster with unsalted butter
DAY 20	Chicken		
DAY 21	Watermelon (if not available, pineapple)		

Week Four

	MORNING	MIDDAY	EVENING
DAY 22	Papaya or kiwi	Hamburger with everything on it *or* tuna-salad sandwich	Fish
DAY 23	Pineapple		Strawberries and 2 glasses wine *or* champagne
DAY 24	1½ Breads	Mini Mazel Salad	Stir-fried vegetables, rice, and sake *or* your choice of any Open Carb meal

	MORNING	MIDDAY	EVENING
DAY 25	Apples		Popcorn
DAY 26	Prunes (8 oz.)	Raspberries or strawberries	Pasta with bread and butter *or* with 2 vodkas
DAY 27	Grapes		
DAY 28	Cherries (if not available, strawberries)		Raisins (8 oz.)

Week Five

	MORNING	MIDDAY	EVENING
DAY 29	Grapes		2 glasses wine *or* champagne
DAY 30	Figs, fresh or dried	Dates (6 oz.)	Potatoes, any style with Mazel or L.T.O. Salad (see recipes, Chapter VI) and vodka, *or* Open Dessert
DAY 31	Mango (if not available, papaya)		Pineapple
DAY 32	Eggs and toast	Mono Protein	Open Protein
DAY 33	Kiwi (if not available, papaya)		Papaya

	MORNING	MIDDAY	EVENING
DAY 34	Pineapple		Mazel Salad and vodka
DAY 35	Watermelon or grapes		

Week Six

	MORNING	MIDDAY	EVENING
DAY 36	Papaya		Pizza, as you like it, *or* Mexican dinner
DAY 37	Pineapple		Strawberries
DAY 38	Watermelon (if not available, grapes)		
DAY 39	Papaya or kiwi		Chinese, Japanese, *or* Middle Eastern ethnic dinner (Mexican and Italian *excluded*)
DAY 40	Watermelon (if not available, strawberries)		

	MORNING	MIDDAY	EVENING
DAY 41	Papaya		Traditional "balanced" American dinner
DAY 42	Pineapple, papaya, mango, strawberries, *or* kiwi		Popcorn (no salt or butter)

V

Tricks of the Trade: Tips, Pitfalls, and Other Secrets

HOW YOU'LL FEEL

The process of Conscious Combining is experiencing food and how it makes you feel. Few people realize that food is energy. Three little grapes, and you're ready to run a mile. Your body is constantly putting out energy and replenishing its supply. The Beverly Hills Diet teaches you how to maximize not only the quantity but also the quality of that supply. By now, you should be well on your way to learning to control how you feel by what you eat. You should be feeling too well to ever dissipate into your bloated, sluggish former self.

So how should you be feeling on my diet? For the most part, you'll feel absolutely marvelous. You will feel an abundance of energy. You'll be able to concentrate more easily. And you'll probably need much less sleep.

By the end of the first week, you should notice a definite change in your skin color. It should glow. Your eyes should begin to sparkle. Your hair should begin to shine. The dark circles under your eyes should disappear. As one client said, "My friends are amazed. They're not only talking about how thin I am, but how young I look! What a fabulous bonus. Your diet is miraculous!"

It's one of the most common comments from my clients. They are always delighted with how well they look. Most other diets sap your body of nutrients, and it shows.

As you lose weight, you won't have that drawn, haggard look we expect to see in a successful dieter. You're losing weight not by starving your body but by feeding it.

Be aware of your energy as you begin reintegrating familiar foods into your diet. Tune in to the effect of pineapple on your state of being. Feel the charge that papayas give your system. Be aware of the relaxing effect of a potato. In other words, tune in and turn on to your feelings. No two foods have exactly the same effect on your body. When you think about it, it makes sense doesn't it? Isn't it logical that different foods affect your energy differently? It's just that you've never been receptive to the process before. You've never let your skinny voice have the floor before. Well, that's what these five weeks are all about—experiencing food.

If you taste a little salt in your mouth on occasion, don't worry. That's old salt leaving your system. You are going to feel clean. You'll feel full. And you won't want to cheat.

Because you're going through a detoxifying process, you may feel a little peculiar the first week. How you feel will depend on how toxic you are. If your recent diet has been high in additives, sugar, and salt, you might have a slight headache—nothing severe. Remember, your body has built up an addiction, and there may be a withdrawal.

While most people feel an abundance of energy, there may be moments when you feel slightly drained. Especially on a watermelon day. How appropriate. . . .

One of the symptoms of hunger is a tired feeling. If you

should feel this, eat more. If you have loose bowel movements, hooray! Keep in mind that pounds leave your body two main ways—bowel movements and urination. The more time you spend on the toilet, the better. On watermelon days especially, you can expect to urinate a lot. That's the idea.

If fruit has given you gas in the past, it's because you've eaten it with other foods. It shouldn't happen now, but if it does, it means old food is moving out. It will pass. No pun intended. . . . Remember, we're breaking up all those fat deposits, and they're going to accumulate and collect before they're pushed out.

Tips for Success

1. Always buy a lot, making sure you have *more* than enough. Never set yourself up to fail by running out of what you need. If you have any left over, you can always cut it up and stick it in the freezer.

2. Don't leave the house for more than twelve minutes without your food. Baggies, Tupperware, and tinfoil are quite wonderful inventions. Avoid being a victim; always have *enough* food with you. You never know when your emotions are going to sneak up and grab you.

There is no reason to be a victim on the Beverly Hills Diet, because this is your diet—a diet *you* control. Think about yourself and what you need. Food has always been important to you; now is the time to make it really important. You, your diet, and your food should be your top priority for these five weeks.

3. Don't share. Everyone will want to eat your food, especially on grape days. Don't let them. Your generosity can get you in trouble. What happens if you run out?

4. Use your imagination with fruit. Try eating some of it with a knife and fork. It doesn't have to be finger food. See "I Bought It,

Now What?" in Chapter VI for some clever ideas on what to do with fruit.

5. If something appears tempting, remind yourself that you only know it tastes good because you have tasted it before, and by the same token you can taste it again. It's not leaving the planet. It will still be here tomorrow.

I was at La Scala Boutique, a restaurant in L.A., on an abysmal blind date; my weight was up; and I was on pineapple. The steaming bread and butter had never smelled so good. I kept repeating to myself, "It's not leaving the planet. The restaurant is not burning down; it will be here tomorrow." It worked. I did not succumb to even a crumb. The next day my weight was down. I went back to La Scala Boutique and ate an entire basket of bread loaded with butter—with permission, with enjoyment, without guilt, *and* without gaining an ounce!

6. If you blow it, don't make it worse by blowing it further. Remember you are not blowing your diet forever, you are only blowing your discipline, and it is only *temporary*. Learn about the corrective counterparts in Chapter VI, and use them.

7. If you can't drink coffee or tea without a sweetener, try putting in some cinnamon or a little piece of the fruit you are on that day. Both are wonderful.

8. Read all labels carefully. Remember that salt, sugar, and additives lurk in the most unsuspecting places.

9. Talk about your diet. Tell the world what you are doing. It's going to be hard to hide it anyway. Watermelons and papayas are not exactly unobtrusive.

You only develop a skinny voice by using it. *Use it now.* If you feel yourself weakening, don't be ashamed to ask for help. Tell someone how you are feeling. I still do.

Getting thin requires developing a support system that is active and alive, one you can call your own. That's one of the joys of my Beverly Hills Diet. We Conscious Combiners are net-working a support system across the country.

Remember, you cannot do it alone. You need help. Yes, even you. Ask for it!

10. Remember this is *your* diet, so build it around the foods you love. On maintenance you're intentionally not getting a list of specific foods to eat for each mealtime. Although this is my program and my methodology, it is *your* diet, and your diet should focus on the foods that you love, not the foods I love.

In Conscious Combining you are learning that what you choose to eat determines what you have to eat so you can have anything you want. The sky is the limit if you are willing to do whatever it takes to make it work. If, for instance, you want to eat pizza, the next morning you will have to eat pineapple. If you plan for it, nothing is fattening. Remember, think about food when it doesn't count so you don't have to think about it when it does.

Physical Exercise

Don't be afraid to do physical exercise during these first weeks. You are feeding your body pure energy. I'm not adding an exercise program to the Beverly Hills Diet, because most of you feel guilty enough to begin with. Why should I give you something else to feel guilty about? Another excuse to set yourself up to fail? Something else you *have* to do that you don't want to do and won't do?

If you *want* to exercise, terrific. All the better. The best things you can do are aerobics—walking, running, and swimming—or yoga. At this point in the diet, the purpose of exercise is really to help you get in touch with your body, to make you conscious of it.

Frankly, the amount of calories you'll burn up is relatively unimportant. But the awareness you'll gain is not. That's the big benefit of exercise, at least at this stage of the losing game.

Don't misunderstand. Firming, stretching, and improving breathing are happy side effects of exercise. But right now, I am most concerned with your consciousness. It is the melding of your mind and body that will make the Beverly Hills Diet work for you forever.

Under no circumstances should you exercise with weights. Building muscles is obviously not our objective. Who wants to build up and compact all that old fat? Before the fat can leave your body, it has to soften up, which is precisely the purpose of those enzymes you have been experiencing. I want you to do everything you can to promote that action, not thwart it.

The Nonphysical Exercises

Nobody said getting skinny was going to be easy—fun maybe, but not easy. Fat does not let go without a fight. It will rear its ugly head at every opportunity. It's spent years staking out and building up its territory, and it will use every resource to protect it. But, don't forget, it can only exist if you feed it.

You will become a thin person by using your thin voice, a voice that has always been a weak, little whisper but that is now becoming a shout—a voice that will outshout the strident, blustering voice of fat. We have to develop that voice.

That's what my nonphysical exercises are all about—to give voice to your skinny soul. You should do the exercises at the end of each week just as scheduled. If they seem silly, if they seem unsophisticated, try them anyway. They are going to help you breathe life into that skinny voice.

Englebert Humperdinck did them. I did them. So did hundreds of my clients. You can do them, too. Let yourself go.

The exercises, just like the rules, are what made me and hundreds of my clients thin. Thin is far more than just eating right. It's thinking right, internalizing that skinny voice forever. It's meshing the mind and body, curing the mind/body split, so you can synergize and focus all of yourself on controlling your energy and feeling your body. Remember, my Beverly Hills Diet is a methodology *and* a philosophy.

As you lose weight, you may find your emotions are being supercharged. You're letting go of feelings. With each pound you lose, you're letting go of unexpressed, unacted upon emotion. The exercises facilitate this process. You become a thin person by feeling and confronting all those emotions that made you a fat person. With each pound you lose, you move to a new place. You literally experience the world from a different vantage point. Acknowledge, confront, experience, and let go.

The Scale

The scale, that little mechanical device that has more effect on us than an atom bomb. It can literally make or break our day. It can take the strongest of egos and shatter it to smithereens. I have seen the most gorgeous, the most powerful, the most secure, and the most self-assured crumble beneath its force. The scale, along with food, represents the enemy. Or should I say represented the enemy?

For most of our lives we have been trying to get away with murder, but we have condemned ourselves to a life sentence. We have been running away from our one link to reality. The one thing that forces us to see what we have been blinded to: ourselves.

The scale forces us to see and feel ourselves as we *really* are, and it forces us to do something about it. Do you think that if you had really seen yourself as you were you would have let yourself look the way you did? If you had *really* felt yourself,

don't you think you would have done something about it long before now? How easy was it to carry that heavy watermelon from
the check-out stand to your car? How easy was it to carry
around all those extra pounds? If you had felt them, if you had
really been conscious of them you would not have been able to
do it.

No matter how evolved we get, how thin we get, we retain
this investment in disconnecting from our bodies, a vestige of our
mind/body split. We see what we want to see, and we feel what
we want to feel. When we look in the mirror we have a preconceived idea of what we look like and *that* is what we see.

My first trip after I had gotten skinny was nine days in New
York City. Nine days without my scale, away from my "Farmers
Market," nine days of being wined and dined. Would Conscious
Combining really work, would it stand the test out there in the
"real world"? I was scared! What a relief, when I arrived at the
hotel, to discover there was a scale in my hotel room. Each night I
celebrated—as a Combiner, of course, eating but following the
rules, and each morning I weighed myself. Conscious Combining
was working. Joy of joys! My weight was a constant 102.

One night, I gave myself permission to really splurge, to do an
Open Human, and I did, in grand style. It was an Open Italian,
and I mixed it all: grease, cheese, and salt—a real "mishamishima." (See Glossary.) I had tried to eat like a mensch but I
was sure I had gone overboard. I was sure I had gained. The next
morning I could feel it as I rolled out of bed. When I looked in the
mirror my hip bones had vanished. I *knew* I had really done it this
time. I was terrified. The whale that I had once been was looming.
I inched onto the scales with dread and horror. With one eye shut,
barely breathing, I looked down. Three numbers stared up at me
—102: I had not gained an ounce! I had succeeded. I had eaten like
a mensch, with one hand, one bite at a time, I had done an Open
Human, and I hadn't gained a pound. I didn't have to be afraid

anymore; I could schedule them in more often. I was overcome with joy and relief, and when I looked in the mirror again, my hip bones had reappeared.

What a sense of security the scale affords! From that moment on I haven't traveled without one. I have a small, very lightweight bathroom scale that slips easily into the bottom of my suitcase.

Your scale is your best friend; it's your nonjudgmental lover. It is the one truly objective observer in your life. It has no ulterior motives. It no longer tells you if you've been good or bad, but rather if what you are doing, what you are eating is working or not working. And if it's not working, if you've gained a little, big deal; it's not the end of the world. It doesn't mean that you should get hysterical and beat yourself over the head at what a fat failure you are. It doesn't mean that you will never again be able to eat whatever it was you ate. It means that you will make it work. That is what the Beverly Hills Diet is all about. Making food, *all* food, regardless of its inevitable and transitory effect, work. So, the scale is up—you'll simply apply the rules of Conscious Combining, use the corrective counterparts (See page 146) and eat your way back down. You got thin by feeding your body, and you'll stay thin by feeding your body.

In Conscious Combining you've been experimenting with food to see what works and what doesn't work. You are learning to make food work for you. Believe me, this can only happen if you commit yourself to a daily love affair with your scale.

The scale is there to tell you exactly how much you can get away with. To define the precise margin for rule stretching. Emotions play an important role in weight loss: the more important food is to you, the more you love it, the higher its price and the less you can get away with. The more emotional my clients are, the less frivolous they can be in their eating.

The worst thing you can do is not weigh yourself after you blow it. Keep in mind that it's not the big meals that get you, it's not the indiscretions you've planned for or those "moments of madness," it's all the things you think really don't matter (the lick off the spoon you stirred with). Let the scale prove it to you. Make it your best friend and your lover.

Every day of your life, confront your weight, acknowledge your weight, and, if you need to, let it go. Every day of this diet, weigh yourself, write it down, and tell it to the same person. Erase that fat consciousness once and for all.

If you don't confront and acknowledge your weight, it hangs around. Here's an example: Jackie used to tell me her weight in code. She'd write down ten pounds less than it was, and when she called her weight in, she'd only give the last digit. She thought her husband, Henry, had no idea of what she weighed. Then she got stuck on a plateau.

Nothing was working. Her weight remained at the same maddening number. Of course, I felt that if she would admit her weight, the plateau would dissolve. Yet nothing could persuade her, not the thought of three watermelon days in succession, not threats, nothing.

Finally, in desperation, I asked her to put her husband on the phone as I had something to ask him. She consented. "How much do you think Jackie weighs, Henry?" Despite her code, despite her dressing in the closet to hide her fat, despite every ploy known only to the fat, Henry guessed Jackie's weight within a pound.

Once Jackie realized that her weight wasn't a secret, and once she herself said it aloud, she lost three pounds. The plateau had been mental, not physical.

Love your scale and embrace it; it is the key to your success and your foundation to your sense of being. It will make this diet work for you, and it will make food and eating work for you. It will get you skinny and keep you skinny if you'll only let it. What have you got to lose?

Pitfalls: The Subtle Subterfugers

The world is out to undermine you. TV ads assault you. A harpie lurks around every corner. Be especially aware of the innocents—your friends. They are the most dangerous of all.

"You're crazy to be on a diet like that!"

"Chocolate ice cream and you expect to lose weight?"

"Oh, another fad diet. . . ."

"You're getting too thin."

"You don't look well."

"It's not going to work. . . ."

Ad nauseum. "It's not healthy," they'll snipe as they eat their hot dogs and salty potato chips and smoke their cigarettes.

The talk-back exercise you learned in Week Five should stop them dead in their tracks.

Don't count on a lot of positive support. As the Beverly Hills Diet starts to transform you, your fat friends will feel intimidated and guilty. Your thin pals won't want any competition.

"Oh. You can have one little bitty bite," they'll insist. No, you can't! One bite throws the whole thing off. I always laugh when I ask a client if she or he "stuck" to the diet and they reply "sort of."

There is no "sort of." You either did it or you didn't. And what's the point of doing it if you're not going to do it right? Remember, it isn't easy to be gorgeous, but it sure is fun!

The Peaks of Peril: Plateaus

Plateaus are those inevitable unannounced places we all reach when the weight loss stops. Day after day, we get on the scale, and no matter how good we've been, we don't get our reward. The scale doesn't budge.

How did we deal with this in the past? By eating, of course. Out of frustration, we'd shove it in. If you can't lose, you might as well gain. Right? Doesn't make you feel too good about yourself, does it?

Maybe, if you understand a little bit about what plateaus really involve, you'll be able to ride them out without the usual anxieties and desperation.

On a purely physical level, the fat has got to get out of your body. It has to be softened and burned before it is ultimately flushed out and eliminated. This doesn't happen in an instant. First, fat leaves the cell. Then it has to travel to the appropriate channel of elimination—the kidneys and large intestine—before it leaves your body. It's not a short, easy trip.

That cell where the fat resides doesn't just disappear. After the fat is gone it fills up with water. It came into being in the first place because there was extra food to be had. The cell isn't leaving. It's waiting to be fed again. Sooner or later, however, it gets the message that you are not going to feed it. Speck by speck, it begins to shrink—and so do you, right along with it.

If you become conscious of this process, if you are doing the mirror exercise, you will realize that while the scale isn't so much as flickering, your body is changing quite dramatically. Hang in there. The water that is gradually leaving the cell will ultimately be flushed out. You never know when a plateau will strike or just how long it will last. Joe hit a plateau on the third day of the Beverly Hills Diet, a time when almost all clients are losing the fastest. Janet's plateau came just before her big trip to Europe, when she wanted to be her slimmest. Fat does not play fair.

During my final weight loss, when I was "going all the way," I got stuck for a full thirteen days at 108 pounds despite desperate measures. Once I had proven to myself that I wouldn't give in to Fat, once I had proven that I would not succumb to the lure of cashews or raisins or anything else I wanted to eat, I began losing again. The following week, eight pounds dropped off.

Plateaus are not only physical but also emotional. In fact,

they are emotional more often than not. Remember the case of poor Jackie, whose weight wouldn't change until she admitted what it was?

Plateaus give us time to catch up with our new bodies. They allow our heads and bodies time to get back in sync. If you have lost, say, twelve pounds, you are experiencing life from an entirely different vantage point.

You don't have the twelve pounds of padding and armor that you once had. You are more vulnerable. And you need to consciously assimilate your new being. Take advantage of plateaus to do just that. In reality, you are a different entity every time you lose a single pound.

All of our lives, we've either been on a diet trying to lose weight or we've been off our diet—which means we're gaining. Do you ever remember just being—neither losing nor gaining? Have you ever simply stopped and said, "This is where I am right now?"

So often we are so obsessed with our final goal, which may be some ten or thirty pounds away, that we don't stop to experience now, to feel today.

This pattern is another example of the mind/body split: that stage when the mind has not caught up with the body. (See page 52.) It is a major cause of plateaus. Plateaus are breathing spaces, a time to mend your mind/body split. If you let them, plateaus can be highly positive. Experience yourself where you are now, not where you've been, not where you're going, but where you are right now.

Says Carol, "I am skinnier and more attractive now, with cheekbones to knock your socks off. The sizes of my clothing are small; the appreciation for the new Carol is great." But, conscious of the mind/body split, she adds, "I can feel the extra bulk I will take off in the not-too-distant future. But I am comfortable and want to assimilate this particular me. That sense of self before I move on to another."

Plateaus give you an opportunity to make a choice. You can ignore your mind/body split and eat. This is what you have probably done in the past, and it is one of the reasons you have been fat. All the frustrations, the anxieties, the hostilities, and the depressions you feel each day as you weigh yourself are only feelings you've had before. Feel them and let them go. You don't have to swallow them anymore. You *know* the scale will move.

By this time you have probably lost about fifteen pounds. That's equal to about seven chickens. (A chicken weighs about two pounds.) Do you feel it? Are you looking in the mirror? Are you doing the nonphysical exercises?

Acknowledge your new body as it is today. When you do that, it will change.

Outlasting a plateau means stating your case and saying "This is forever. I will do whatever it takes. I want to be thin more than anything, even food." Once you are willing to give up *anything*, there's only one thing you will have to give up—and that's FAT.

Before you can choose not to be fat, you have to understand what makes you fat. Only then can you rid yourself of it and become thin.

Plateaus make you confront that fat person, and they force your hand. This is the test. Are you *really* committed? Are you willing to go the distance? Do you have what it takes to be skinny? My Beverly Hills Diet and Conscious Combining give you all the tools you will ever need. Use them.

You do have what it takes, you know. You have proved it by coming this far. So just give it up and let it go—your fat that is.

Welcome slimhood!

Overcoming Old Habits

1. Nibbling. Don't be a victim. As the late Totie Fields used to say, "It flew into my mouth!" What difference does a bite make? Plenty. It affects the whole digestive process. Don't so much as lick the crumbs off your fingers when you cut your son's peanut butter sandwiches. Each and every bite is important. Remember, think about food when it doesn't count, so you don't have to think about it when it does. When food isn't feeding your heart and soul, then it better feed your body. There is nothing out there you cannot eat, if you plan for it.

2. When visting a friend in the hospital, don't take a box of *your* favorite candy.

3. At bridge club, don't serve *your* favorite danishes. Don't cook your family *your* favorite miscombinations, if you haven't given yourself permission to eat them. Don't set yourself up to fail.

4. Always have your food available. If you are used to eating popcorn at the movies, be sure to take some of whatever you happen to be eating that day with you instead. Or go to the movies on a popcorn night.

If you love to eat on the phone, if you can't fall asleep on an empty stomach, or if you are used to waking up in the middle of the night and raiding the refrigerator, have your food right there with you.

5. If you can't resist leftovers, have someone else clear the table—and the plates.

6. Be aware of unconscious eating. While complaining to me that she wasn't losing, the wife of a famous comedian swore she wasn't drinking diet soda anymore. At the same time, she crossed to the bar refrigerator, pulled out a Tab, and began drinking unconsciously. Hers is not an uncommon problem. Watch yourself, carefully.

7. If buffets are your downfall, avoid them.

8. If you expect to be perfect, to never blow it again, you are setting yourself up to fail. Part of what this is all about is giving yourself permission to blow it—"Blow It Without Blowing It," that is.

9. Eat and chew slowly. Experience it. See how long you can make the pleasure last. You don't have to inhale it, you don't have to see how much you can get in in how short a time. You have permission to eat and enjoy it.

Excuses I Have Heard

There exists in the eater a constant struggle between the skinny self and the fat self. When the fat self wins, when the old diet consciousness reasserts itself and takes over and the heart smothers the intellect, we pile on the excuses, hoping to bail ourselves out. Don't do it. You're wasting your energy. You are catering to FAT. Stop and think. Use your head.

After all, anything can be rationalized. Any flimsy excuse will do if we want it to. You've been using excuses long enough. That's one of the main reasons you're fat. The luncheon meetings are not going to end. All the restaurants will not burn down. Dinner parties will still be thrown thirty years from today. Your social calendar will never be clear. And your emotions are not leaving. They will always be poised to throw you off balance at the barest provocation. I know.

- Your boss yelled at you.
- You got fired.
- You got promoted.
- You need an operation.
- You had an operation.
- Your mother yelled at you.
- Your mother baked a cake.

- Your boyfriend didn't call.
- Your boyfriend did call.
- You're going on vacation.
- You're bored.
- You're tired.
- You're nervous, upset, miserable . . . ad infinitum.

Manufacturing excuses is probably the easiest exercise going. Because it's escaping.

You're going through a separation? Well, so was Bill Blount. He not only lost twenty pounds, but he also stopped smoking. All between Thanksgiving and Christmas.

You've already paid for the big benefit dinner? Lorimar Production's Irwin Molasky took his watermelon to Joe Louis's benefit in Las Vegas.

Friends are visiting from out of town? Rita (Mrs. Jerry) Vale gave a dinner party, and as each of the nine gourmet Italian courses were presented, she ate a delicious fig. Neil Bogart, record executive, did the same—with his watermelon.

Barry wakes up every morning with good intentions. He's on the racquetball court at 6:00 A.M. He follows his diet slavishly—until each afternoon, when his intentions vanish as the pressures build. As he builds his excuses right along with the pressures.

Carol's excuse is always "I have to cook for my family." She has used this excuse twenty-two days out of thirty.

It's funny. We reward ourselves with food and we excuse ourselves with food. Whether we have been good or bad. It really doesn't matter. In either case, of course, the reward becomes the punishment.

My clients are very creative when it comes to excuses.

"A fly flew on my fingernail, and I had just had a manicure."

"My papayas got cockroach spray on them."

"Instead of watermelon, I ate gazpacho. . . . Well, it was red, like watermelon."

Anything will do. . . .

Karen had made it. She was down to a size six. "People were raving," she said. "I had never been so thin. So I ate."

Rejecting Your Skinny You

Letting go of the fat image and the fat consciousness comes with time. It comes from knowing that the thin person is here to stay because you have a way of eating that ensures it, that allows you to turn to food in your moments of madness without food turning on you.

You can be your own worst enemy. If you expect to be perfect, to never blow it again, you are setting yourself up to fail.

You love to eat, you live to eat, and it's been killing you. It is a conflict that, until the Beverly Hills Diet, you haven't been able to resolve.

You've hidden from it. You have sneaked food. You have denied your enjoyment of it in your eagerness to "please" yourself and those around you. This constant denial of what you are has only made you what you don't want to be—fat.

Why try to shut the mouth of an eater? Use it and embrace it. Once you've given yourself permission to eat, your love of eating won't hurt you anymore. You will gain control.

Thin people have permission to eat happily. So do you. It is guilt that works against you. Guilt is an emotion of the heart. Enjoyment is an emotion of the intellect. The fat consciousness is glutted with guilt, laden with regrets and "if onlys" and "to-morrows." Fat comes from the heart, skinny from the head.

Nobody expects you to be perfect in your eating behavior. Except you. Stop dwelling on the negative. Work back through the nonphysical exercises. In the process of becoming a thin person, you will learn what made you a fat person. Don't feel guilty. If you do blow it, don't heap even more blame on yourself. Accentuate your positive qualities. Accentuate the times you didn't blow it, all those times you resisted the temptation.

So you made a mistake. Big deal. Think about all the times you didn't make a mistake. Don't dwell on the negative. Stop interfering with your innate developmental process, your transformation into a Combiner, into a Skinny. Stop judging yourself and start living.

Cheating

If you plan for it, nothing is fattening. You can plan for everything, so why would you cheat? I know. . . .

On my five-week Beverly Hills Diet, each day follows another for a very specific enzymatic reason—to complement, augment, or embellish the processes already under way. If you should cheat, heaven forbid, *do not continue with the diet as outlined.*

Instead, refer immediately to the corrective counterpart section of Chapter VI. Follow the plan specifically and carefully, taking into account the type of mistake you made and the amount of weight you gained. Once you have completed that plan, then go back and pick up my diet where you left off.

Obviously, it's faster, easier, and much more fun if you don't cheat.

But if you do, don't forget that once you've blown it there's always something you can eat that will make you feel better and lessen the blow. That's one of the miracles of this diet. It takes into account the human being in all of us.

Don't feel guilty. It's never too late even once you've blown it. It isn't the first time you have cheated, and it won't be the last. Who are we trying to kid?

One client, Jerry Gold, liked the all-fruit days so much, he'd blow it on purpose. But you will probably not want to follow his lead.

We all get crazy. We eaters are feelers. We know that. But there is that moment of clarity when we can again begin to make conscious choices. That is the time to use the corrective counterparts.

My Beverly Hills Diet is not like other diets. There are no nevers. If being back on the diet meant you could never again have the foods you love, you would have good reason to cheat. With the old fat consciousness, you're never going to eat those foods again, so you might as well cram them all in, because it really does become the "last supper." Three little chocolate cupcakes expand into a hamburger with everything on it and a hot-fudge sundae. Before you know it, you are trying to cram a lifetime of foods into that single moment.

Since there are no never-again foods on my diet, why binge?

Running out of food or not having food with them is the reason most people give for "cheating." I repeat, *always be prepared.*

Expecting Miracles

Don't. It's the old syndrome of setting yourself up to fail. You didn't gain your weight in a day. How can you expect to lose it in a day? If there were a miracle to be had, I promise you, I would have unearthed it.

The only miracle there is in losing weight is finding a discipline you can stick to—the Beverly Hills Diet.

The magic pill hasn't been discovered. Rather, the magic is in your soul. It's that skinny voice waiting to be nurtured and set free—forever. You are doing it; that's the miracle.

VI

Maintenance:
Getting Away with Murder
Without Serving
a Life Sentence

Welcome to the world of the little golden pineapple. Isn't it glorious? Now you move from thin to skinny. Your transition from temporary to forever. That's what my Beverly Hills Diet and Conscious Combining are all about.

One of the things that makes people stay thin is experiencing the high of getting on the scale and honestly saying "I do not have to lose one more pound!" As long as you have weight to lose, if it is one or one hundred pounds, the world is filled with foods that you cannot eat, because you have to lose weight and they could be fattening.

Once you are perfect, you have your choice of *anything.* You can eat whatever you want. Once you have no more weight to lose, you no longer have to deny yourself anything. Gone is the "I can't have it; it's fattening, and I have to lose five pounds or three pounds or even one pound" syndrome. You don't have to lose anything so you can have anything. It's funny that most of the things we want, we only want because we can't have them. Once we can have them, we realize we can have them anytime we want them, they will always be there, and having them right now is no longer important. What becomes really important is maintaining our state of perfection and the freedom that accompanies it.

Now, for the first time in your life, you are in control. You have let go of that fat consciousness that screams "Feed me! Feed me!" No longer does that voice dominate your world.

No longer is that the last voice you hear when you go to sleep at night and the first voice you hear in the morning. Fat is no longer crowding out the rest of the world. Your energy and your power are your own. You are free.

Have you noticed that when you control your eating, the rest of the world falls into line?

Have you noticed that your power is no longer scattered and diffused? That you are no longer totally consumed with thoughts of food and eating and dieting?

No longer are you your own worst enemy. No longer does the universe whisper behind your back "He's fat!" or "She's fat!" Now you can do anything. You're looking gorgeous. You're feeling great. And you're even eating ice cream! That old consciousness, the anxieties and insecurities caused by being fat, the neuroses, hating yourself, never enjoying the food you were bolting—they're all vanquished. Isn't it wonderful not to be ashamed of eating anymore? Not to be ashamed of yourself anymore?

Now you are ready to begin living and making choices. Choices based on eating what you really want, not what you think you *should* want. It's going to be fun. Because you've made the biggest choice of all—the choice to be thin.

What you choose to eat will now determine what you have to eat. The foods that really matter to you will now become a part of your life. On a practical level, and remember this is a methodology as well as a philosophy, you will look forward to a pineapple day almost as much as to a hamburger with everything on it. Not only because it tastes and feels great, but without that pineapple, you know there's no way you will ever be able to enjoy your hamburger without guilt and fear.

You have given yourself permission to make food the most

important thing in your life. And, because you have, food has become less important. Once and for all, it has been put into proper perspective.

You no longer feel deprived when you don't have that sumptuous patty melt or that loaded submarine. You know you can have it tomorrow. What now makes you feel deprived is not being able to fit into those size seven slacks.

Now you can go to bed every night feeling good about yourself. Now you can experience the freedom of getting up each morning without having to decide which diet to go on. Now you can keep your eyes open when you pass the mirror. Now you have given away or burned every fat outfit in your closet. Now that you can dress in front of the mirror and make love with the lights on, is it really that difficult to wait and make choices? Now that you have learned how to have your cake and eat it too, what difference does it make if you have to eat it one piece at a time? You have learned that nothing is leaving the planet—except your fat and neuroses. What possible excuse could you have for ever getting fat again?

I still love to eat. I still live to eat. I always will. When food is in my mouth, my heart sings and my soul soars. But there's at least one thing I have come to love even more than eating: buying clothes in a size four.

I am still obsessive and compulsive when it comes to food and eating. I still eat a triple order of potato pancakes without choking, an entire roast beef without blinking an eye, a whole, extra-rich cheesecake without a single gasp.

I still respond to emotional situations by eating. So can you. When I awaken at night, I still make a beeline for the refrigerator. But, when my heart says go and my head says no, I dwell on the joys of my wonderfully lean hipbones and make choices.

If I can do it, if I can maintain, so can you.

STRETCHING THE RULES

Although no two bodies handle food in exactly the same way, the basic physical laws are the same for everyone. As I said earlier, every time you miscombine you will not gain weight. Otherwise, you'd weigh at least three hundred pounds.

So how do you figure out how much you can get away with? Each person's capacity to stretch the rules of Conscious Combining is different. The most important factor is your relationship to food and the role it plays in your life.

The more important it is to you, the more it usurps your energy and your power, the less you can get away with. I, for example, get by with very few transgressions.

At the other extreme, Jackie Applebaum, our Beverly Hills lady, has a terrific tolerance. She had gained weight to begin with not because she was compulsive, but because of the good life, fabulous restaurants, and fancy dinner parties. Now the good life has gotten even better. She's thin again. She's in control.

Maintenance means experimenting—experimenting without fear. What's the worst that can happen? You'll gain a pound or two. That's a necessary part of your learning process. Some foods will be harder for your body to digest than others. Maintenance is all about seeing what works and what doesn't work for you as an individual. This is *your* diet. You're taking my rules and creating a diet, a way of life for yourself—forever.

If something doesn't work, if you gain weight when you eat it, if it turns out to be fattening, you are going to learn how to make it work. How to make it *less* fattening by counteracting or negating its negative side effects, the extra pounds your scale showed you picked up. That's the purpose behind Conscious Combining. That's what separates the Beverly Hills Diet from all other diets. You don't have to give up the things that don't work—you make them work.

Corrective Counterparts

By this point, you should have glorified and solidified your love affair with your scale. (See page 128.) Your scale should be almost as important to you as food. Remember, your scale doesn't reward or punish you. It simply tells you what works and what doesn't work. Now, more than ever, it is critical that you continue to weigh yourself each day. The scale is the single most important tool for achieving eternal slimhood.

If something isn't working, you will gain weight. But, let's face it, some days, you'll be up. Others, you'll be down. Don't panic, and don't revert to the old fat consciousness of "My God, I'm doomed. I'm fat. . . ."

A weight gain means you have not digested, not yet processed what you ate the day before. The reasons vary: it could be salt or the combinations of what you ate, or it could even be your state of mind. For every hard-to-digest food, there is a *corrective counterpart*, something that will help digest it.

It was the enzymes in the fruit you ate that caused your weight loss during my five-week diet. Now you are going to see how those same enzymes will help you maintain that weight loss.

Eat the appropriate corrective counterpart on the day following a weight gain as follows:

AFTER GREASY, CREAMY, OR
CHEESY FOODS SUCH AS: BURN WITH:
French fries   Pineapple
Lobster newburg
Spareribs
Creamed spinach
French meals
Mexican, Middle Eastern, or
   Italian meals

Ice cream
Cheesecake
Quiche

AFTER PROTEIN SUCH AS:	DIGEST WITH:
Beef	Papaya
Turkey	
Chicken	
Veal	

AFTER SWEETS SUCH AS:	FEED WITH:
Candy	Grapes
Pie	
Sweet rolls	
Mousse	

AFTER SALTY FOODS SUCH AS:	WASH WITH:
Chinese food	Watermelon
Deli food	
Salty fish, lox, or herring	

AFTER OVERDOSING ON	UNPLUG WITH:
Maxi Carbs SUCH AS:	Prunes (8 oz.), Strawberries,
Bread	or Raisins (8 oz.) for the
Potatoes	entire day. Be sure it is a carb
Pancakes	overdose, not an overdose
	of what went with the carb
	(the butter, or the cheese,
	or the sugar).

How much of the corrective counterpart you will eat the following day will be determined by your best friend, the scale.

Don't think of eating as traditional mealtimes of breakfast, lunch, and dinner. Think of eating as food experiences separated by two- or three-hour increments.

To simplify matters, I have broken the day into three parts, just as I did for the diet. You can manipulate those parts in any way that satisfies you, day by day, if you are so inclined, as long as you observe the time divisions of two or three hours between eating experiences. I personally break my day up as follows: from the time I get up until 1:00 P.M.; 3:00 to 5:00 P.M.; and 7:00 P.M. to bedtime. Your own schedule will dictate how you break up your day.

In using corrective counterparts, you can apply them to one-third, two-thirds, or to your entire day. Again, the added poundage recorded on your scale will determine how much of your day to devote to it. You have no choice. Your scale chooses for you. When you have the choice of eating anything at all, you have to relinquish some decisions. What you *choose* to eat now determines what you *have* to eat.

If your weight has not changed despite what you ate, you don't have to do anything other than breathe a sigh of relief. You must have behaved like a human being, not a fat person. Skinny people don't gain every time they eat, because they know when enough is enough. You must have, too. And you proved it.

But if, despite your most serious effort, you did go a little crazy, and your scale is up as follows:

¼ to ¾ pound	Begin the day with the appropriate corrective counterpart.
¾ to 1¾ pounds	Eat the appropriate corrective counterpart for two-thirds of the day.
More than 1¾ pounds	Eat the corrective counterpart for the entire day, please.

Follow this plan until you have zapped the extra weight. All of it. Don't be surprised if it takes more than a day. Some of us pay a hefty price for our indulgences.

Recoups for Special Meals

Your scale will tell you whether the following special recoups are needed. Perhaps the simpler corrective counterparts listed above will do. Or maybe you're lucky like Cindy Griffith, who can eat Open Mexican meals and not gain an ounce.

These special recoups are to be followed for one, two, or three days. You should never need more than three days to recoup.

FOR	*Open Mexican, Open Italian, Pizza, Thanksgiving dinner, Christmas dinner,* or *Open Human.**
DAY 1	Pineapple and Papaya
DAY 2	Papaya and Pineapple
DAY 3	Watermelon

FOR	*Open Oriental* (AND THE HIGH-SODIUM CONTENT THAT AFFECTS US BLOATERS)
DAY 1	Watermelon. If you are still up, do the next two days.
DAY 2	Pineapple and three bananas
DAY 3	Watermelon

---

* Remember that "Open" means anything. The above are considered to include a "mishamishima": grease, sugar, salt, the works.

Conscious Combining involves not only knowing what does and does not go together, but also knowing what counteracts what. With the Beverly Hills Diet, you have a remedy, and you know how to use it. Remember, I took some simple physical laws and synthesized them into a diet—one that can work for you forever.

But remember, too, that I promised no magic. In order to maintain, you are going to have to plan in advance for what you want to eat. As I will explain more fully later in this chapter, it's best to work out your eating schedule a week at a time.

Keep in mind that your diet should be made up of about 50 percent carbs, 30 percent fats, and 20 percent protein. And be aware that the more fruit you eat, and the fewer miscombinations, the more likely you are to lose or maintain your weight.

Daily Combinations for Maintenance

I am going to outline the kinds of daily combinations you can put together to maintain your weight. I am listing them in order of their weight loss or maintenance potential, with the least "fattening" first and the most "fattening" last.

First, here are the symbols I use, defined:

F = Fruit

C = Carbohydrates, or Carbs

P = Protein

OF = Open Fruit

OC = Open Carb

OP = Open Protein

(Refer to Chapter III for a complete definition of the different food groups as well as a complete listing of each.)

For a complete explanation of the different types of meals, see page 88 in the introduction to Week Four of my diet.

MO = Mono Meal
 A single protein, a single carb, or a single fruit.

OF = Open Fruit
 Combining fruit with wine, champagne, or brandy.

OC = Open Carb
 Combining three carbs at a single meal with no more than two being maxi carbs. (see Chapter III for list)

OP = Open Protein
 Combining three proteins, excluding nut proteins.

OM = Open Miscombination

1. One carb and one protein. Eating the carb first.
2. *An entity unto itself.* A carb and a protein combined in one dish. Entities unto themselves, such as quiche, pizza, spaghetti and meatballs, sandwiches, and casseroles.

OH = Open Human
 Eating a traditional meal in moderation, with any combination of carbs and proteins. Eating like a "mensch," with one hand, one bite at a time, and watching a skinny person and mimicking him or her.

RO = Resnick Open
 Drinking instead of eating.

OD = Open Dessert
 Two human portions of any dessert at lunch. Three portions of any dessert at dinner.

On maintenance, don't feel you have to make every meal a Mono Meal. Although that is how they are shown in the list that follows, you'll get bored. Don't deprive yourself. Conscious Combining is fun! So remember, depending on your week and how much entertaining you are planning, you can turn any of the carb, fruit, or protein meals into Open Meals.

In the following outlines, the first letter represents the food designated for the morning, the second letter represents the food to be eaten during midday, and the third letter represents the food to be eaten during the evening. In the example F C P, you eat fruit during the morning, carb during midday, and protein in the evening.

Under each combination, I have listed several examples to clarify the possibilities for you. Use your imagination! Include your favorite foods and don't forget that any Mono Meal can be converted into an open meal.

Here is the list of daily food combinations for maintenance and examples of each:

F F F   Pineapple/Strawberries
Pineapple/Papaya
Prunes/Strawberries/Raisins
Watermelon

F F C   Strawberries/Mazel Salad
Prunes/Raisins/Baked Potato
Mango/Pineapple/Pasta and Salad (F F OC)

F C C   Pineapple/Salad/Stir-Fry Vegetables
Papaya/Vegetables/Pasta

F C P   *Note:* For those still worried about the "balanced meal," this is the perfectly balanced day. This is how you, as a Beverly Hills Diet maintainer, should eat most of the time. It is the kind of a day you should strive for in your planning.
Pineapple/Salad/Steak

            Strawberries/Steamed Vegetables/Lamb Chops
            Prunes/Vegetable Tempura/Shrimp Cocktail
            and Lobster (OP)

F F P   Mangoes/Cashews
            Pineapple/Strawberries/Steak and Lobster (OP)

F P P   Papaya/Hamburger/Chicken

P P P   Eggs/Chicken
            Steak/Chicken-Liver Omelette/Fish (P OP P)

F F OM   Strawberries/Hamburger with everything on it
            Pineapple/Papaya/Steak and Salad

F F OH   (Here's the difference between Open Human and
            Open Miscombination in action.)
            Strawberries/Hamburger with everything on it,
            french fries, and a Coke
            Pineapple/Papaya/Steak, Salad, Vegetables,
            and Wine

F OM P   Pineapple/Corned Beef Sandwich/Chicken
            Strawberries/Spinach Omelette/Seafood

F OH P   Pineapple/Corned Beef Sandwich with Potato
            Salad and Cream Soda/Chicken
            Strawberries/Spinach and Mushroom Omelette,
            Toast/Seafood

OM P P   Eggs and Toast/Fish/Steak
            Bagel and Cream Cheese/Plain Omelette/Veal

OH P P   Bacon, Eggs, and Toast, Coffee with Cream
            and Sugar/Fish/Steak
            Lox, Bagel, and Cream Cheese/Plain Omelette/
            Veal

The examples given are foods that blend well together. They are like little family units. Don't forget, any straight Mono Meal can be turned into an Open Meal, *depending on what your scale tells you.* If your weight is constant don't be afraid to experiment. See for yourself how much you can get away with.

THE MEANS TO MAINTENANCE: RESPECTING THE RULES

The Fixed Rules

1. Once you have gone off fruit in the course of the day, do not go back to it. Do not eat fruit again until the following day.

2. Nothing follows protein on any day except more protein. Once a drop of protein has crossed your lips, be it cream cheese on that bagel, cream in your coffee, or bacon in your salad, you are locked into protein. Note that the sample days with OM and OH always follow the protein rule. If you follow this rule, you will never get fat again.

3. Watermelon and grapes are the only all-day fruits. Once you begin eating them, you must continue with them for the entire day.

Their enzymatic action is very specific, and the time it takes for the enzymes to work varies. On some watermelon days, for example, you'll urinate instantly. On other days, it might be delayed for several hours. *If you block their action by adding other foods, you'll probably gain weight.*

The General Rules

You might be lucky and be able to stretch these general rules; don't be afraid to experiment with them a bit. They are for the typical Conscious Combiner.

1. A dried fruit should never be eaten the meal before or the meal after (including breakfast the following morning) an animal

protein. It digests so rapidly that it will meet the still uneliminated wastes from the protein in your large intestine and cause gas.

2. Nut proteins, including avocado, only end all-fruit days. They do not combine well with other proteins, either at the same meal or on the same day, regardless of the order in which they are eaten. Avocado combines with nothing but itself and a little lemon juice.

3. Maxi Carbs (*see* Chapter III *for a full listing*) should never be eaten the meal before or the meal after a protein. Examples: Don't have pasta for lunch and steak for dinner; don't have steak for dinner and English muffins for breakfast the following day.

4. When you know that later in the day you will be eating an Open Human or an Open Miscombination, keep your eating light. Keep yourself "enzymatically open." A fruit day is ideal. The antidote, the corrective counterpart, is also effective as a "precidote." (*See* Glossary.)

5. In open meals, although you are not required to, it's ideal to stay in the same family of foods—fish with fish, eggs with chicken. Remember that your energy comes from the foods you eat and different foods generate different kinds of energy. Upon seeing someone eating "a surf and turf" (steak and lobster), I remarked to my friend "his body won't know whether to sink or swim."

6. Limit yourself to one Open Meal a day. The mouth of an eater is like a finely tuned piano. Each little bite brings out a different note, and we're only happy when those notes are playing in harmony.

7. Neutral fruits, such as apricots, nectarines, peaches, pears, and plums, can be eaten any time you don't need a corrective counterpart. They can also be used as "precidote" to an Open Meal.

8. At this stage of the game, you have learned whether or not you are a bloater. And you have learned how to deal with it.

If you are like me, highly sensitive to salt, you avoid it assiduously. If you're lucky, like Linda Gray and Pat Harrington, you can get away with some salt. Even if you can, do not use salt voluntarily. Never add it to foods while cooking or eating them. But you do not have to special-order foods, nor do you have to avoid Chinese restaurants or go on two watermelon days after eating in them. Your scale will be your guide.

9. Pineapple is the closest thing to a panacea I have discovered. If you are ever in doubt as to what corrective counterpart to apply, turn to pineapple.

10. Don't go on a watermelon day or a grape day after something greasy or if cheese has been involved. You will bloat. Use pineapple.

11. Use rice vinegar (a carb) in salad dressings instead of wine vinegar (a fruit). Salad dressings can be either oil and vinegar or sour cream, garlic, and rice vinegar, loaded with fresh herbs. (See recipes.) The sour-cream dressing is added on maintenance and should *not* be eaten during the weight-loss period.

12. Make cheese a special occasion. Treat it with respect. It is the hardest food to digest, and it contaminates everything you eat it with. Eat it only as the last meal of the day, and even then, only on rare occasions.

13. If you are on a protein night, you can pick out and eat the protein when it is mixed with other foods and not interfere with your digestive process.

You cannot do the opposite—that is, eat the carb and leave the protein. The carb will not make the protein indigestible but the protein will make the carb indigestible, hence—fattening. Take a vegetable beef stew. The odds are that it has a chicken- or beef-stock base. If you are on a protein meal, pick out the meat and leave the vegetables. Their mere presence won't affect the digestion of the protein.

However, if you are on a carb meal, you cannot eat the vegetables. Protein will have entered the very soul of that innocent little carrot and rendered it indigestible. If you eat the vegetables, they'll get clogged in your stomach while the protein you didn't even really eat is being digested.

14. Continue to avoid diet soft drinks. They are awash with chemicals and sodium.

15. As for drinking, remember what goes with what. Champagne, wine, and brandy with fruit. All other liquors, including beer, with carbs. Nothing with protein. Again, you'll need to see what you can get away with and what you can't, what works for you and what doesn't.

Don't be awed by all the rules and guidelines. Each feeds into the next. They are easy to assimilate, even easier to practice. As director James Sheldon so articulately expressed, "Out of the confusion comes practical clarity, and after you stub your toe a few times, you learn to walk with great ease. The personal pride in the way you feel and look makes it easy to say no to your hostess and yourself."

Your objective is to make them habit.

You now have the keys to eternal slimhood. Use them. What could be more rewarding?

The Most Dangerous Maintenance Foods and Combos

1. Sugar and salt are probably the worst of all.

2. Meat and potatoes eaten together because both are hard to digest.

3. Carbonated beverages. They cause bloating because of their naturally high sodium content.

4. Adding cheese to a carb meal. In light of the consequences, how important are a few grains of salty parmesan on your pasta? Use fresh-ground pepper and fresh chopped parsley.

5. Adding proteins to carbs
6. Cheese on anything
7. Milk in your coffee

Keep in mind that milk is a protein, and all it takes is a drop of protein to throw everything off. When you start your car, it doesn't matter if you turn it off right away. The engine still has to gear up, whether for a second or an hour. The same applies to your digestive system. Either one drop or one pound of protein ignites your enzymes.

Everything in the Beverly Hills Diet comes down to you as an individual, your particular tolerances. Linda, one of my clients on maintenance, talks of the fun of "slowly finding out what foods I digest well and those I don't. Fruit, of course, is perfect. Steak is O.K. . . . Strange that I lose on a day of carbs and gain on a day of fish."

Says Bill, "I get extra pleasure out of eating, because I'm not paying for it in pounds or heartburn." He talks of the pressures to conform to traditional eating patterns. "For the first time in my life, I've thrown away my Rolaids, yet everybody tells me I'm wrong. There is no sense in doing things to make other people happy if I'm the one to pay the price for it."

Milton exulted when "for the first time I chose not to have the chocolate soufflé at The Bistro. I knew I could have it any other time I wanted to."

Says Mary, a successful maintainer who knows that cheese does her in, "If I'm going to gain three pounds, I'm going to appreciate it. I'll bury myself under mounds of mozzarella." Everybody works out their own system. They take my rules and apply them to their diet.

The following guidelines will help you to maintain. But first go back, and if you haven't already, memorize the commandments and rules that precede the Beverly Hills Diet in Chapter IV. They are vital to your success as a Conscious Combiner. Know them, understand them, and internalize them.

Charting Your Weekly Slimhood

Now that you have achieved your goal, and I don't say that lightly, but with great exuberance, rather than thinking in terms of your daily weight, think in terms of your weekly weight. Start whenever it suits you. Sunday to Sunday. Tuesday to Tuesday. Remember, Beverly Hills Dieters are thinkers, not sheep. Your mind should always be on your diet.

From one week to the next, your weight should be the same. It should never fluctuate day by day more than three pounds above your ideal. Remember, if you plan for it, if you schedule it in, nothing is fattening.

Since you probably know your business and social schedule a week in advance, it's best to schedule yourself by the week.

Make a weekly chart for yourself and fill in all your commitments first, the things most important to you.

My schedule often looks something like this.

Monday:	Business lunch at The Hamlet
Tuesday:	Business lunch at the Bistro Garden
	Chinese dinner party at the Feldman's
Thursday:	Dinner party at the Donahoe's, menu unknown
Friday:	Business lunch at The Palm
	Dinner at Ma Maison
Saturday:	Cocktail party at the Applebaum's
Sunday:	Brunch with the Blauner's

I'll plug those commitments into my week's chart first and then build the rest of my eating plan around them.

My goal: not to gain a single pound.

The Beverly Hills Diet
Weekly Chart

	MORNING	MIDDAY	EVENING
MON.	Strawberries	The Hamlet hamburger with everything and french fries	Chicken
TUES.	Papaya	The Bistro Garden strawberries	Feldman's Open Chinese
WED.	Watermelon		
THURS.	Pineapple ——————→	Mr. Chow's	Donahoe's OC, OM, or OH
FRI.	Papaya	The Palm steak, salad, and cheesecake	Ma Maison poached salmon
SAT.	Grapes ————————————————→		Applebaum's champagne

	MORNING	MIDDAY	EVENING
SUN.	Blauner's lox, bagels, and cream cheese	Chicken	
MON.	Watermelon ————————————————————→		

MONDAY 102 pounds. Strawberries will enzymatically set me up for the greasy hamburger and french fries at lunch. Remember, the enzyme in strawberries promotes hydrochloric acid, the fat-burning agent in your stomach.

Chicken follows because I had protein for lunch. Because I have eaten protein, I must stick to protein.

TUESDAY 103 pounds. I'm up a pound from Monday—from the salt in the catsup, the grease in the french fries, and possibly from too much protein. I'm digesting with papain in the papaya, burning with the berries—a good choice in a French restaurant because they are nearly always available. I usually eat three orders of berries, by the way.

To compensate for the extra pound, I eat fruit for two-thirds of my day today. I also want to keep myself enzymatically open for the Chinese dinner. I don't want to limit myself to anything. I think about food when it doesn't count. I don't want to have to think about it when it does. Diane is known for her Chinese cooking.

WEDNESDAY 104 pounds. Well, I did it. I didn't handle my Open Human like a human. Everything was just too good. The salt-ridden soy sauce really got to me, and I'm up two pounds from my ideal weight. So it's watermelon all day today. If I had any social commitments today, it wouldn't make any difference. I knew the consequences of an Open Human might be a weight gain. Now is the time to correct it, not next week. I know my social life isn't going to wither and die.

Not long ago I ate only baked potatoes at the Scandia Restaurant, determined to immediately lose the pound I'd gained the day before. Lucky I did. Because a long-lost love appeared in town and took me to Jimmy's the next night.

THURSDAY   102¾ pounds. I am still up three-quarters of a pound from the Chinese food, and I have no idea of what the Donahoe's are having for dinner. I don't want to lock myself into a choice ahead of time. Plus, I want to lose that three-quarters of a pound. I take my pineapple with me and give it to the maitre d' at Mr. Chow's, where I'm having lunch with a business associate.

Will Mr. Chow's get upset? I'm a good customer, and they know I'll be back and spend money. The maitre d' gladly accepts it and charges the minimum. It's one of my favorite restaurants. Oh well, I know I can go back tomorrow.

At dinner that night, I choose Open Carb because the entree is oversauced, oversalted chicken breasts. How boring. Dessert is a nondescript mousse. No sacrifice there.

However, there is a lovely salad, delicious bread with unsalted butter, and a wide array of crudités. Much to my delight, Ceil serves artichokes vinaigrette as an appetizer. My choice is easy.

FRIDAY   102 pounds. My weight is where it should be! Lunch at The Palm is so wonderful I stick with my decision to go Open Human and indulge. To get myself ready for the basically high-protein meal, I have papaya in the morning for its enzymes.

I am proud to say I eat my lunch like a human. With one hand, one bite at a time. I even leave some on my plate. Just because something is good doesn't mean more is better. I know I can go back anytime I want to.

I have oil and vinegar salad dressing. Remember, fats combine with anything. Although I would prefer roquefort, why add insult to injury? Roquefort is loaded with salt.

Because I had protein for lunch, my dinner choice at Ma Maison is obvious. And I adore their salmon.

SATURDAY   102 pounds. My weight is fine. I didn't gain an ounce. I'm going on a fruit day today, not because I gained weight, but because I want to drink wine tonight and not have my weight be up tomorrow for my brunch. The only safe combo with wine or champagne is fruit. I choose grapes because I know I want to eat a lot today. I am going to have a hectic day, the grapes are easy to carry around with me, and I can nibble to my heart's content. Plus, the grapes at this time of the year are glorious.

SUNDAY   101 pounds. Even though the salt in the lox will make me bloat, it won't matter. I have that special security that only comes from being under my ideal weight.

At the Blauner's brunch, it's hard to resist the delicate miniature pastries heaped with all the things I love. To reward myself for not succumbing, I have an extra lox and bagel. Not exactly deprivation. Later that day, I eat an entire roasted chicken.

MONDAY   102¾ pounds. My body simply won't tolerate extra salt. That lox is a killer. It's watermelon for me again today to flush it all out.

P.S. It worked. On Tuesday I am 102 again. Another week of freedom from fat.

You will notice that just because I can't tolerate salt, I don't banish it from my life. Your body may tolerate salt better than mine. I made choices that week—choices based, above all, on staying thin. Today, I can't even remember what I gave up last week. All I know is that I am still thin. And I don't feel deprived.

It may sound complicated. It isn't. Weekly meal planning and Conscious Combining really become second nature with a little bit of practice and this book for reference. It's easy. It's flexible. And it works.

VII

Your Grocer Isn't God: Conscious Combiners Go Shopping

Many of your meals are Mono Meals, especially during the initial phase of the Beverly Hills Diet. If that single food is not the best, then you are not going to be happy. Eaters are wanters. Why not buy the best when you most need it? At the time you most deserve it?

While you are on the five-week plan, relinquish control over your eating to me. You need waste no energy on deciding what to eat, how to eat, when to eat. Instead, focus your attention on one thing—finding the best Beverly Hills Diet foods available.

When Marty called and told me he couldn't find any pineapple at his neighborhood market, I pointed out that he drives ten miles one way for his favorite pancakes and much farther for his favorite ice cream. "Why," I wanted to know, "can't you give finding a pineapple the same effort?" Marty was actually looking for an excuse to blow his diet. When you shop, make an effort. What could be more important?

When you buy a steak or chicken, you select it yourself, because you know what you are looking for. Take the same responsibility with your fruit. Just because someone works in the produce section doesn't mean he is an expert on produce. After reading this chapter, you will probably know more than he does. Watch out for produce people pushing overripe or overstocked fruit.

If you go to one market regularly, tell the produce man in advance what you need. Most are happy to order it for you. Offer to buy papayas or mangoes in bulk for a discount. I buy my papayas this way and get a 10 to 20 percent discount. The foods on my Beverly Hills Diet are more readily available than you might think. Toni Lopopolo found herself in Emporia, Kansas, on the first week of her diet, and she was able to get *every* first-choice fruit.

HOW TO BUY

Fruit

1. Always buy enough. The worst that can happen is you'll freeze it for those out-of-season days.

2. Don't buy unripe fruit in advance, hoping it will ripen by the time you need it. You will be sorely disappointed. If fruit is not ripe, it means the nutritional potential has not been developed, and it won't taste good.

3. Don't buy fruit that's already been cut unless you're going to eat it the same day you buy it. The nutrients escape, the enzymes dissipate, and the flavor seeps out.

4. Look for a fruit store that doesn't refrigerate its fruit in an attempt to prolong its life. Refrigeration masks fruits' delicate aroma, so it's harder to decide whether it's ripe.

5. Look for premium fruit. Go to the best stores. The best produce is selected and sent to these stores. When you compare the costs of eating this way compared to your old way, you will inevitably find the figures tally in favor of the Beverly Hills Diet— even when you eat the best. You are no longer paying for pack-

aging, preparation, and processing. Plus, you cut out a lot of restaurant expenses.

PINEAPPLE   It should be golden blond on the outside, with darkened, dusty points. Smell the pineapple on the bottom, and if it's sharp and acrid, don't buy it. It should smell sweet and rich like canned pineapple. If it's hard and green on the outside, or if only the bottom part is ripe, reject it. Unripe pineapple will make your mouth sore.

When you cut open a pineapple, it should be a translucent golden yellow inside. If it's white, it's not ripe. It it's brown, it's fermented.

PAPAYA   Perfect papaya is yellowish orange and brushed with green on the outside. In some seasons, it turns yellow. Look at the stem. If there is a tiny yellow ring around it and the papaya smells sweet, it's ripe. Papaya should give to the gentle pressure of your thumb. If the smell is overpowering, or if it caves in to the touch, it's overripe. Underripe papaya is hard and dark green.

MANGO   Because there are so many different varieties of mangoes, you can't always judge them by their cover. Mexican and Floridian mangoes start out green and wind up splotched with gold and red. The midsummer variety of these mangoes should be as golden and red as you can find them. At other times, the skin usually stays green. The Caribbean mango, a flat, kidney-shaped variety, usually stays green. As with all other fruits, no smell, no taste.

There are countless varieties of mangoes, each with their distinctive flavor, inner color, and consistency. There should always be a little bit of give to the skin. If a mango is perfectly ripe, it can be the most exquisite taste you have ever experienced.

KIWI These furry, brown creatures from Australia and New Zealand taste like little green Chuckles candy to me. Don't put the skin to your mouth or your lips will swell. Kiwis should be moderately soft and pliable to the gentle prodding of your thumb.

PERSIMMONS As the last mango leaves the planet, the persimmon appears, just in time for Halloween. It's sweeter than sugar. Unless it's soft and mushy, you'll wind up with a mouth full of fur. Persimmons are always orange and should almost fall apart when you touch them. It's often difficult to find them ripe, but the cupboard-ripening method (see page 169) works like a charm.

BANANAS Remember, the enzymes don't work to capacity if the fruit isn't ripe. Your bananas should be soft and speckled with brown and have a rich, banana-cake aroma.

WATERMELON The trickiest of all. Because of its thick skin, it's hard to tell what lurks inside. We all know how disappointing a lousy watermelon is. Unless it's your watermelon day, resist the temptation to buy it already cut.

Although good things come in small packages, such is not the case with watermelon. The bigger, the better. A little watermelon was stunted in its growth. To test for ripeness, roll it over to expose its belly, the lightest, sun-shielded spot on which the melon has been growing and resting. Look first for little brown worm holes, a sure sign that something good hides within. Fear not; the worms can't get in.

Next, knock the watermelon on its belly with the knuckles of your closed fist. If the sound is a high ping, it's not ripe. If it sounds deep and mushy, it is. Listen for a resounding, not too high, not too deep, solid thump. Experiment with a few side by side. You'll soon become an expert.

Don't try the new seedless variety. The seeds, you remember, are the focus of the nutrients, the storehouse of the enzymes and essential for elimination.

GRAPES   Seedless grapes are tricky, too. If they're too green, they'll be tart. Select those that are turning slightly yellow. They will be richer and sweeter. My favorites are green grapes that are a whisper away from being a raisin.

FIGS   The odder and more shriveled looking the fig, the better it's going to taste. A shriveled, black exterior produces a majestic, purple interior. The plumper and smoother on the outside, the grainier inside. The green variety, when ripe, has a slightly yellow hue around the bottom. Biting into a fig can be one of the most sensual pleasures known to man.

PRUNES   Don't forget to soak them first. Eat them with the pits in. You don't eat the pit, but if the pit's soft enough to bite through those seeds inside are wonderful. But don't break any teeth trying to get at them.

RAISINS   My favorite—the richest and the plumpest—are the Monnuka. They're available unsulphured, of course.

APPLES   Any color will do. And you know the rest. Try to get them unwaxed.

Buy It Ripe

Try to buy only ripe fruit, because you can never trust unripened fruit to ripen according to your schedule, if at all. Of course, ideally you would buy your fruit every day. But, once it's ripe, most fruit will cheerfully stay that way indefinitely in your refrigerator. So you are quite safe buying your fruit a week in advance.

I've had perfect papayas on hold for as long as two weeks. Apples and grapes are typically held in commercial cold storage for as long as six months, so a week or so more will not offend them. Pineapples have a wonderfully long refrigerator life, too. But remember that if you buy any of these fruits too ripe, their fermenting process will continue even if they're refrigerated, and fermented fruit is wine. I know I have said you will get high from this diet, but this isn't what I had in mind.

Unripe, If You Must

If nothing you want is ripe, but fresh is available, you can try ripening it in two ways.

Have the sun do it for you. This is my first choice. Place your fruit outside, unless it's bitter cold, and then put it indoors by a window.

Or put it in a brown paper sack, and tuck it away in a closed cupboard. There are fruit-ripening contraptions at the market or in gourmet-cooking stores that work about the same as the brown bag, closed cupboard technique. One of the best places to ripen fruit is in a glass-fronted cupboard. My first experiment with mangoes, which I'd expected to take days to ripen, was a twenty-hour success. This is a wonderful technique for ripening persimmons, which are often quite difficult to find as soft and as ripe as they should be.

If Not Fresh?

Fresh is preferable to frozen and dried. If frozen or dried is all that's available, by all means buy it instead of substituting another fruit. Substitutions should be made only as a last resort.

Under no circumstances should you buy canned fruit. Even if

it doesn't have sugar or another sweetener in it, salt and a variety of additives will inevitably have been used in the canning process.

Freezing Fruit

If you have a big freezer, cut up your fruit, put it in plastic bags, and pop it in the freezer for those off-season days when you may need it most. Home-frozen berries, for example, are a vast improvement over commercially frozen ones. You can even stick whole watermelons in the snow, where they will happily wait several months for you to eat them.

Dried Fruits

To avoid fruits saturated with sulphur dioxide, which blocks the detoxifying they do, buy them at a health-food store. Unopened, the packages will last indefinitely. Put any leftover opened fruit in your refrigerator, where it will last a long time.

Nuts

Your almonds must have the skins. Don't forget where the nutrients live. For the most taste, buy whole nuts rather than pieces. If you want to make a little extra work for yourself, buy your nuts in the shell.

If you buy nuts in sealed plastic, they'll stay fresh forever. Once opened, keep them in an airtight container.

Cold-Pressed Oil

This can be bought either at a health-food store or in the health-food section of your grocery store. It will be labeled either "cold pressed" or "expellor pressed." Once it's opened, oil should be stored in your refrigerator.

You'll be happy to know that cold-pressed oil comes in all flavors—sesame, corn, olive, safflower, etc.

Unsalted Chips

These are available at your health-food store. By the way, I really have no financial interest in health-food stores, nor am I trying to turn you into a health-food fanatic.

The quality of your energy is, however, directly contingent on the quality of the food you eat. The first step on my road to slim-hood and the creation of the Beverly Hills Diet was the discovery that for every unhealthy food, there is a healthy equivalent.

I was so hooked on Jays potato chips that I'd beg and bribe my friends to bring some back from Chicago every time they went there. I must confess that the unsalted variety at my backyard health-food store is every bit as wonderful.

Raw, Unsalted Butter

Alta Dena is available at health-food stores.

As you may guess, when I shop my first stop is always the health-food store.

Vegetables

Always buy them fresh, if you possibly can. Buy frozen vegetables only when desperate, and avoid canned like the plague.

I BOUGHT IT—NOW WHAT?

I am concentrating on fruits in this chapter because not only are they the core of your diet, but they are probably the foods with which you are least familiar.

· Try eating your fruit with a knife and a fork. It doesn't have to be finger food. Lop off the top of your pineapple and eat it whole with a knife, fork and spoon.

- Stick your fruit in the blender with a little ice, and make a frappé out of it.
- Don't cut up all your fruit in advance; the flavor dissipates.
- Pop those little grapes into the freezer, and eat them as if they were miniature popsicles.
- Go European and make fruit soup. Add a little water and cinnamon, and gently simmer.
- Bake that pineapple as if it were a roast. Or pop the whole papaya into the oven and bake it for about five hours at 125°. Sprinkle with cinnamon and nutmeg. Never cook any fruit at a temperature over 150°, because the heat will destroy its precious enzymes.
- On your watermelon day, snack on watermelon seeds.
- Although it's fine to blend your fruit, don't put it in a juicer because you will lose all the cellulose, the fiber that cleans out your body.

Juices

I have intentionally excluded juice from the Beverly Hills Diet. It's the fruit minus its essential fiber, again an example of man's meddling. Without the fiber, there's nothing to push the waste out with.

Don't forget that juice is overly concentrated calories and without that cellulose. It is food out of balance and I don't recommend it.

The way food makes contact with your mouth makes a difference in how it is going to taste. The fruit hits your mouth in a different place depending on *how* you eat it. You activate different taste buds when you eat with a fork than when you eat with your fingers. Try really chewing your fruit. The fruits you are now eating are far more than snacks. Treat them with respect.

There is an infinite variety of ways to enjoy your fruit. I often eat mine with a knife or a fork. One client cuts a little cap off the top of his watermelon and scoops out its insides. Recording executive Neil Bogart gave a seven-course dinner party, and for each course he had his watermelon served differently—in balls, wedges, and squares. For the main course, he was served half of the melon, and for dessert he was presented with a frozen watermelon frappé.

The point is to think about and feel what you are eating. By eating unconventionally, you are bypassing the unconscious nibbler in yourself in favor of the Conscious Combiner. You are reinforcing your food consciousness.

Eating on the Job

Cut up your fruit, and throw it in some plastic containers or plastic bags. You'll be amazed how simple it is and how much time it saves. The messiest fruit, yes, even a mango, is much less sloppy than a hamburger oozing over the sides of its bun.

Prepare yourself for a lot of attention. "What are you on today?" your friends will want to know. And they will want some.

If you have to drive a great deal, and eating and driving is your thing, you'll be in heaven on the Beverly Hills Diet. I can peel and eat a mango while driving a standard shift car wearing a white silk dress—without spilling a drop. But you don't need to go that far. Keep in mind that this is your diet, designed to fit into your life, not vice versa. Its adaptability is already legend.

VIII
Recipes for Success

Almost any recipe can be adapted to Conscious Combining simply by eliminating the salt and applying any pertinent Beverly Hills Diet rules.

Think of the following recipes as a sampling, as a starting point for your own creations. They are not intended to be an inclusive compilation. After all, this is an eating book, not a cookbook.

Conscious Combining hinges on knowing not only what doesn't go together, but what goes together best. These recipes illustrate some optimum combinations to maximize your energy and minimize your size. The combinations are like little family units designed to feed both your body and your soul.

The Mazel Salad, for instance, is rich in vitamins A and C, potassium, and calcium. The L.T.O. is the perfect balance of potassium, sulfur, and chlorine.

You will find a few of the dishes in the six-week Beverly Hills Diet program. Others can be used when you have Open Carb opportunities. I have not included any protein recipes, because I'm sure you have your own favorites, and there is a plethora of books devoted to them.

By now, you should welcome the fresh, clean taste of pure food. You don't miss salt any longer, and you can probably tell when sweeteners or chemicals have been added to your food. Most people, with the exception of Conscious Combiners, have no idea what a potato really tastes like. Or zucchini. Or pasta. You will find that using garlic and fresh spices like ginger will enhance the flavor of almost everything.

I'm not trying to turn you into a vegetarian. But you may find that you much prefer your Open Carb meals to Open Protein meals.

Many of your favorite recipes combine protein and carbs. If you experiment a little, you will find that the protein adds nothing to the flavor. It merely represents a texture. And that if you omit it, you won't miss it. The only thing you'll miss is the extra pounds you would have piled on from the indigestibility of the carbs.

A big advantage to the Beverly Hills Diet is that you don't have to prepare any special foods. Almost any recipe can be adapted easily and flavorfully to Conscious Combining just by thinking about the rules and following them. Happy eating!

Recipe Notes

All vegetables should be fresh and of the very finest quality.

Dry all vegetables carefully before sautéing or stir-frying; water will cause them to steam. They should also be dried if they are to be tossed uncooked with egg-yolk-only mayonnaise or dressing, which water will dilute and make runny.

To skin chili peppers, char the peppers well under the broiler, then place them in a damp towel for five minutes. Remove the skin under running water, but *use caution*—the seeds inside the peppers are extra hot!

Leeks are so loosely structured that they must be cleaned

carefully. Slit them open and clean every layer separately. Grit is not a sensuous texture.

Clean mushrooms by wiping them with a paper towel or by washing with a little water. If you use water, be sure to dry them immediately with a paper towel; otherwise, they may become soggy.

Shitake mushrooms, on the other hand, must be soaked in water. But use warm water only; hot water tends to make them bitter.

Carrots and other such vegetables should be well scrubbed, but do not peel them; many valuable nutrients lie close to the skin.

Cooked tomatoes should not be peeled because the peels aid in digestion.

You may substitute dried herbs for fresh, but they will not produce the same results. Herbs are fun to grow, and since most are used in relatively small amounts, it's practical to grow your own. They can be preserved in rice vinegar for use in winter; in the tarragon used for Mazel Hollandaise, the vinegar flavor of the preserved herb is delicious.

Wherever the term "whisk" is used in the following recipes, it means to beat with a wire whisk (available in gourmet or hardware stores, and sometimes even in food markets; the best whisk is one made of stainless steel, for it can be washed in the dishwasher).

To peel a garlic clove, gently flatten it by hand or with a knife; the peel will then release readily. Cut off the end and discard any green parts, as they tend to be bitter. Browning also makes garlic bitter, but I'm among those people who like it that way.

If you miss the flavor of salt in any dish, try adding more fresh chopped herbs and garlic to make up for the lack. Freshly ground pepper is also a big help in this respect. And be certain to buy peppercorns in a store where there is a fast turnover of this product; stale pepper has bite but no flavor.

When I use the term "to taste" in the recipes, I mean exactly that. I have tried to be as specific as possible about the amounts of ingredients used, but even if we all liked, for instance, the same intensity of garlic—which we don't—garlic may differ in intensity from one variety to the next. For this reason, it is important to be familiar with the distinctions among different varieties, to know how long your finished product will sit before it is eaten (during which time the flavors will intensify accordingly), and then to decide how much of a certain flavoring agent you wish to add. And, of course, what you want to "star" in your dish may change with your mood. I, for one, like tons of garlic—for me, too much is never enough.

It's important to know approximately how much oil to use for frying. If your pan is heavy and well seasoned, you can cook with less oil. If the oil is hot and you refrain from adding too many ingredients to the pan at one time, you can get away with using less oil. Try to start with less oil than the recipe calls for, and add more only if you need it to keep the food from sticking to the pan. For Mexican flavoring, use corn oil; for Italian, olive oil.

The cooking times given are only suggestions because of the variables involved: the size of the pan, the way the pan heats, the temperature of the food, etc. Experimenting will be your best guide.

DRESSINGS AND SAUCES

Mazel Dressing

¼ cup rice vinegar
1 cup sesame oil
Chopped garlic to taste*
(1–2 small cloves)

Chopped or grated ginger to
taste*
Freshly ground pepper

Combine all ingredients.

YIELD: 1¼ cups.

* From clove to clove and root to root, garlic and ginger may differ in intensity. If they are left to steep in dressing, their flavors will intensify. Therefore, depending on when you make the dressing, on the strength of the garlic and ginger, and, of course, on personal taste, the amounts used may differ. Start with one clove garlic and 6 or 7 gratings of ginger and increase to 3 times that amount if desired.

Mazel Cheese, Mexican or Italian

---

6 onions, peeled and thinly
sliced
¼–½ cup corn or olive oil
(corn oil for Mexican
flavor; olive oil for Italian)
1–2 garlic cloves, minced
½ cup chopped cilantro (for
Mexican)

¼ tsp. dried oregano (for
Italian)
1 tsp. chopped fresh thyme,
or ¼ tsp. dried thyme (for
Italian)

Cook onions in ¼ cup oil, adding more oil if onions start to stick to pan and dry out. Cook until soft and cheeselike. If using medium heat, you can stop cooking after 20 minutes; on low heat, keep going for 45 minutes or longer. Stir every few minutes and *don't burn.*

FOR MAZEL CHEESE MEXICAN   Add minced garlic and cilantro at end of cooking time.

FOR MAZEL CHEESE ITALIAN   Add minced garlic at end of cooking time, plus the oregano and thyme.

---

*Mazel Mayonnaise**

---

1 egg
1 egg yolk
¼–½ tsp. dry mustard (use
   more or less to taste)

3 tsp. rice vinegar
2 cups sesame oil

In a small bowl, whisk together egg, egg yolk, mustard, and vinegar. Whisk in ½ cup of the oil, 1 tablespoon at a time, whisking thoroughly as you go to ensure emulsification. Add remaining oil in a thin stream until mixture is thick and smooth. May be thinned with water.

YIELD: approx. 2 cups.

You can also prepare this mayonnaise in a food processor or blender.

VARIATION   Add chopped garlic, pepper, or fresh herbs. If you are using a processor and want to add herbs, chop them in the processor before making mayonnaise and blend them in at the last minute. Or leave them in while making mayonnaise to produce green mayonnaise. Good herb choices, depending on the

---

* If this is to be combined with a carbohydrate, substitute an extra egg yolk for the whole egg to keep the mayonnaise a fat. When made with a whole egg, it becomes a protein.

season, are tarragon, basil, thyme, dill, parsley, chives. Use about ¼ cup chopped herbs per recipe, if fresh, and 1 tablespoon, if dried.

---

*Mazel Hollandaise**

---

1 Tbs. cold water
4 egg yolks
2 sticks unsalted butter, cut
    into small pieces and at
    room temperature

1 Tbs. rice vinegar
Cayenne and pepper to taste

Beat yolks and water together over low heat[†] for a moment in a heavy aluminum pan. Gradually add butter, raising and lowering pan so that the mixture does not get too hot. When all butter has emulsified, add vinegar and seasonings.

Pour mixture into a small thermos or hold over warm—*not hot*—water (Hollandaise does not need to be piping hot to be good; what you're serving it on can be hot.) If held over hot water, the Hollandaise is very likely to separate. If this should happen, add a teaspoon or two of boiling water, whisk madly, and pray!

YIELD: 1½ cups.

* This is classified as a fat, and can be combined with a carbohydrate or a protein.
† Hollandaise is traditionally made in a double boiler, which is fine if you are new at it. However, once you have learned to make it directly over the heat, you will find the cooking time goes much faster.

Mazel Marinara

4 tsp. olive oil
1 cup finely chopped onion
½ cup finely chopped carrot
2 tsp. fresh basil or pesto
  (p. 187)
4 tsp. finely chopped parsley
½ bay leaf

2 lbs. fresh tomatoes,*
  coarsely chopped
1 Tbs. tomato paste (salt-free,
  of course)
Freshly ground pepper
Hot red pepper flakes
  (optional)

Cook onions in oil till translucent. Add carrots and cook 4 minutes. Add basil, parsley, and bay leaf; simmer 2 minutes. Add tomatoes, pepper, and tomato paste, and simmer 30 minutes. Add red pepper flakes, if desired.

YIELD: 3 cups.

* You may want to peel tomatoes for some dishes, such as pizza, as the peels definitely change the texture of the finished dish.

Hot and Spicy Salsa Mazel

1 large onion
2 Tbs. corn oil
6 cloves garlic
2–6 fresh chili peppers*
8 large tomatoes
2 Tbs. parsley

2 Tbs. cilantro
6 fresh chili peppers
2 fresh jalepeño peppers
  (Optional—eliminate
  jalepeño to make it less
  hot.)

* As a precaution, wear gloves when handling chili and avoid touching your eyes. These peppers are hot little devils.

Sauté onion in corn oil for 3–4 minutes. Soften but do not brown. Mince garlic and add to onions. Mince and add chilis. If fresh chilis are not available, substitute 2 Tbs. dried red chili. Sauté mixture an additional 1–2 minutes, but do not brown. Chop tomatoes and add. Sauté 5 minutes or until salsa is to desired thickness. Take off heat and add parsley and cilantro.

YIELD: approx. 2 cups. The longer you cook it, the smaller and hotter the amount you get.

Note: the smaller the chili, the hotter the taste.

Fresh Mexican Salsa

8 large tomatoes, coarsely diced

1 large onion, peeled and finely chopped

2 cloves garlic, peeled and minced

2 Tbs. chopped parsley

2 Tbs. chopped cilantro

1/4–2 tsp. chopped jalepeño chili

Combine all ingredients and toss gently.

YIELD: 5 cups.

SALADS

Mazel Salad

2 bunches spinach, thoroughly
   washed
2 bunches watercress
2 small heads Belgian endive
1–2 bunches mustard greens
3 carrots, grated
2 raw beets, grated

Daikon radish, grated
25 mushrooms, cleaned and
   sliced
1 bunch chopped parsley
3 leeks cut on diagonal in
   ¼-inch pieces
Mazel Dressing (p. 178)

Be sure all vegetables are clean and thoroughly dry. Tear spinach, watercress, endive, and mustard greens into large, bite-sized pieces. Toss all with Mazel Dressing.

YIELD: 2 servings.

Mazel Slaw

1 large green cabbage, grated
4 carrots, grated
1 bunch scallions, sliced
   diagonally

Mazel (egg-yolk) Mayonnaise
   (p. 179) or Mazel Dressing
   (p. 178)

Combine vegetables. Gently toss with desired dressing to serve.

YIELD: 2 servings.

Mini-Mazel
---

2 bunches spinach, washed
   thoroughly
20 mushrooms, cleaned and
   sliced

3–4 large leeks, cleaned and
   trimmed carefully
Mazel Dressing (*p.* 178)

Combine vegetables. Toss with dressing to serve.

YIELD: 2 servings.

The £-J-O
---

1 large, firm head iceberg
   lettuce
4 tomatoes
1–2 cucumbers, peeled

1 large red, or Spanish, onion,
   peeled
Mazel Dressing (*p.* 178) or
   olive oil

With a sharp knife, cut all vegetables into good-sized chunks. Toss with desired dressing to serve.

YIELD: 2 servings.

PASTA WITH PLEASURE (P-W-P)

Buy fresh pasta, if possible, or make it yourself.

It is important to buy good quality dry pasta, as the taste and texture will be much better. Health-food stores have whole wheat pastas, and my favorite brand, which is carried in Italian grocery stores, is De Cicco, made with semolina and imported from Italy. Do not buy pasta made with soy flour or salt.

If pasta is fresh, leave at room temperature, uncovered, for one day or freeze it. Some pasta shops sell pasta which is refrigerated; they will advise you on how long it can be kept.

Cook according to package directions; though I suggest bringing about 6 quarts of water to the boil for every 1 pound of spaghetti. Add a dash of oil and cook at the boil to the *al dente* stage, which means "to the tooth," or still chewy. Some people suggest throwing a strand of spaghetti against the wall; if it sticks, it's done! Cooking time will vary with the thickness of the particular cut of pasta. Usually it takes about 8–10 minutes.

Drain and toss with desired sauce. I prefer not to rinse pasta with cold water unless I am baking the dish later or letting it cool. Some people, however, prefer to rinse it.

Pasta with Olive Oil and Garlic
(agli e olio)

1 lb. spaghetti, fettucine or linguini
½ cup olive oil, plus oil for cooking water

2–3 large cloves garlic, peeled and minced
Freshly ground pepper

Cook pasta in several quarts of boiling water with a few drops of oil. Cook to *al dente* and drain thoroughly.

Heat oil and toss in cooked pasta. Cook 1–2 minutes over medium low heat. Toss in garlic* and cook 30 seconds over low heat. Do not brown garlic. Add a few grindings of fresh pepper.

YIELD: 2 servings.

* Some cooks recommend sautéing the garlic in oil first; if you do sauté it, use caution and don't brown it, or it will be bitter. Cook only until slightly golden; then add to pasta.

Pasta with Butter and Garlic

1 lb. spaghetti, fettucine, or
   linguini
1 tsp. oil
½ cup (1 stick) unsalted
   butter

2–3 large cloves garlic, peeled
   and minced
Freshly ground pepper

Cook pasta in several quarts of boiling water with the 1 tsp. oil. Cook to *al dente* and drain thoroughly.

Heat butter in a large skillet but do not brown it. Toss in pasta and cook 1–2 minutes on low heat, or just until pasta is hot. Toss in garlic and cook 30 seconds. Add fresh pepper and serve.

YIELD: 2 servings.

Pasta with Sautéed Vegetables

8 large mushrooms, cleaned
   and sliced
½ cup, plus 2 Tbs. olive oil
10 broccoli flowerettes,
   blanched 2 minutes and
   refreshed†
10 asparagus spears, cut
   diagonally, blanched 2
   minutes and refreshed†

1 lb. spaghetti, cooked and
   drained*
2 large cloves garlic, minced
Freshly ground black pepper

* Some people cook the pasta in the water the vegetables have been cooked in.

† "To refresh" means to rinse under cold water.

Sauté mushrooms in 1 tablespoon hot oil for 1–2 minutes. Set aside. Sauté broccoli one minute in 1½ teaspoons hot oil. Sauté asparagus one minute in 1½ teaspoons hot oil.

Heat ½ cup oil. Sauté pasta 1–2 minutes. Add vegetables and garlic and cook one minute. Add pepper and serve.

YIELD: 2 servings.

Pasta with Peas

---

1 cup onions, finely chopped
¼ cup butter
¼ cup olive oil
2 cloves garlic, finely chopped
10 ounces small pasta shells, cooked and drained

6 ounces large pasta shells, cooked and drained
2½ cups cooked peas
1 cup parsley, finely chopped
Freshly ground pepper

Sauté onions in combination of butter and oil for 6–8 minutes. Add garlic and cook very slowly for another moment or two. Remove from heat, add shells, peas, parsley, and pepper. Mix well to serve.

YIELD: 2 servings.

Pesto Sauce for Pasta Dishes

½ cup parsley, preferably Italian, stems removed
¾ cup basil (must be fresh), stems removed
4 cloves garlic, peeled and trimmed

½ cup olive oil
Freshly ground pepper
Sufficient liquid reserved from cooked pasta, after it has been drained, to thin pesto to sauce consistency

Purée all ingredients with mortar and pestle or in food processor or blender. Whisk reserved liquid into pesto and toss pesto with pasta.

YIELD: ¾ cup.

Lasagna

---

1 lb. lasagna noodles, cooked, drained, and rinsed in cold water
1–2 onions, chopped and sautéed in 2 Tbs. butter

30 mushrooms, sliced and sautéed in 3–5 Tbs. butter
1 recipe Pesto Sauce, at room temperature (*see p. 187*)

Layer noodles, onions, and mushrooms in baking dish (you will probably want 3 layers of pasta and 2 layers of vegetables). Drizzle layers with a bit of Pesto Sauce. Bake uncovered for 25 minutes at 350°. Spoon on remaining Pesto Sauce to serve.*

YIELD: 2 servings.

VARIATION 1   If you prefer more vegetables in proportion to the pasta, try adding sautéed zucchini, broccoli, or spinach to the mushroom layers.

VARIATION 2   If you wish, you may substitute 1 recipe Mazel Cheese Italian (*p. 178*) for the chopped onions. You will then have more onions in the lasagna.

---

* Vegetable lasagna is delicious, nutritious, and a boon if you are entertaining, since it can be refrigerated after being prepared and then baked whenever you are ready to serve it.

POTATOES—ANY STYLE

Baked, french fries, cottage fries, of course.

HOT POTATO   Bake, split open, and season with lots of grated fresh horseradish root and cayenne.

BALDWIN SKINS   Bake potatoes, scrape out pulp (use for something else), and rub skins with butter. Sprinkle with cayenne and black pepper and crisp lightly under broiler.

AMERICAN POTATO SALAD   Boil, peel, and dice potatoes, and dress with chopped scallion, chopped celery, chopped red peppers, and onions that have been sautéed in oil and cooled. Toss with Mazel Mayonnaise (made with egg yolk only, *p. 179*) to serve.

ITALIAN POTATO SALAD   Boil, peel, and dice potatoes. Sauté chopped red and green peppers in olive oil. Toss potatoes and peppers with additional olive oil, crushed fennel seeds, and finely chopped garlic. Serve warm. If you wish, add pepper and chopped herbs.

Use Pesto Sauce (*p. 187*) on baked or boiled potatoes.

Potato Latkes 1

---

4 large unpeeled potatoes,   1 Tbs. unsalted matzo meal
   finely grated   Freshly ground pepper
1 onion, peeled and finely   1/4–1/2 cup safflower oil
   grated

Rinse potatoes and onions, but do not soak. Grate them and squeeze out liquid. Add meal and pepper and toss gently to combine. Allow to sit 1–2 minutes so that meal will be well moistened. Form into pancakes.

Fry pancakes in small amount of hot oil till brown and

crunchy on both sides, pressing them now and then with a spatula. Test first cake for doneness. Depending on size, latkes will have to cook about 4–5 minutes on each side.

YIELD: 2 servings.

Potato Latkes 2

1 small yellow onion
3 large russet potatoes
2 Tbs. potato flour

Unsalted butter or safflower oil
Sour cream topping (*optional*)

Grate onion and potato. Add flour, and form into pancakes. Fry in unsalted butter or safflower oil.

YIELD: 2 servings.
VARIATION   Omit the onion and use sour cream/cinnamon topping.

Sweet-Potato Fry

2 sweet potatoes or yams
4 carrots, scrubbed
2 leeks, thoroughly cleaned
2 Tbs. safflower oil

Cinnamon and nutmeg
2 bunches spinach, thoroughly
   cleaned

Cut sweet potatoes thinly on the diagonal. Cut carrots a bit thicker, also on the diagonal. Cut leeks on the diagonal, using the white part and a bit of the tender green part.

In hot safflower oil, stir-fry the potatoes, carrots, and leeks till brown and crunchy. Cover and cook till they are just tender

(10–15 minutes).* Season to your taste with cinnamon and nut-meg. Cook uncovered until crisp again.

Uncovered, toss in spinach leaves until they wilt, not more than a few seconds.

YIELD: 2 servings.

VARIATION   Use unsalted butter instead of the safflower oil.

SOUPS

Gazpacho

4–5 large tomatoes	6 Tbs. olive oil
½ cucumber	3 Tbs. vinegar
½ green pepper	½ tsp. black pepper
1 slice onion	⅛ tsp. cumin seeds

Using blender or food processor, blend together tomatoes, cucumber, green pepper, onion, oil, vinegar, black pepper, and cumin seeds until soup consistency is obtained. Chill. Serve with diced tomatoes, cucumber, and green pepper, as condiments.

YIELD: 2 servings.

* Time will depend on the thickness and quality of the vegetables, and on how well done you like them.

Spinach Soup

---

2 bunches of spinach, washed
   and drained
1 potato
1 carrot

1 slice onion
3 cloves garlic
Parsley or cilantro
Cayenne

Chop or use food processor; then boil in water.

YIELD: Approximately 4 cups.

OPEN CARB COMBOS

Couscous Mazel

---

8 shitake mushrooms
1 large onion, finely chopped
1 bay leaf
2 Tbs. sesame oil
3 garlic cloves, finely chopped

1 tsp. cumin powder
Cayenne
Dill weed
1 cup cooked couscous (see
   cooking directions below)

Soak mushrooms in warm water till soft (about 15 minutes).
Squeeze out water and discard hard stems. Cut mushrooms into
small pieces.

Sauté onion with bay leaf in sesame oil till soft. Add garlic,
mushrooms, and spices, and sauté till onions are a bit brown.

Mix all ingredients together with cooked couscous. Remove
bay leaves before serving.

YIELD: 2 servings.

To cook couscous:

1 Tbs. sesame oil	1 cup couscous
1 bay leaf	2½ cups water

Heat sesame oil in pan. Add bay leaf and couscous. Brown lightly, being careful not to burn.

Transfer to a pot with 2½ cups of water. Boil until water makes little volcanic gurgles. Lower heat to its minimum, cover pot, and steam till water is absorbed (15–20 minutes).

Mazel Pizza

Dough:

1 cake yeast	1 Tbs. crushed fennel seed
1 cup lukewarm water	1 tsp. crushed, dried red pepper
1½ cups unbleached flour	flakes
1½ cups whole wheat flour	
4 Tbs. olive oil plus 2 tsp. to
grease bowl	

Crumble yeast into water and stir.

Place flour in mixer (entire dough can also be made by hand) and add yeast mixture and 4 tablespoons of oil. Dough should be soft, but not sticky; if necessary to get the proper consistency, add a bit more flour or a bit more water. Add fennel and pepper flakes, then knead dough till smooth and elastic.

Put 2 teaspoons of oil into a clean bowl, plop in dough, and flip to grease it all over. Cover bowl with plastic wrap and place in a warm place (about 80°) to rise till doubled (about 1–1½ hours).

Filling and Baking:
Preheat oven to 500°.

2½ cups good olive oil
1 cup extremely thick Mazel
   Marinara *(p. 181)*
7 large onions, sliced thin, with
   slices separated
2 red bell peppers, sliced
1 green bell pepper, sliced
20 fresh mushrooms, sliced
   thick
1 Tbs. crushed fennel seeds

1 Tbs. crushed, dried red
   pepper flakes
14 Italian plum tomatoes,
   peeled, seeded, and juiced
9–10 large garlic cloves, peeled
   and minced
3 Tbs. mixed fresh herbs (2
   tsp. dried) such as parsley,
   thyme, chives, oregano

Cook onions in 1½ cups oil on low heat for 40 minutes or until they are very soft.

Divide dough into 3 parts for baking in 3 separate pans (9-inch omelet-shaped pans are perfect; however, if you have only one oven, you will need pans without handles). Place 3 tablespoons of oil into each pan. On a floured surface, roll out each piece of dough into a thin circle. Roll edges, pressing them to make the outer edges thicker than the bottom of the dough circle. The bottom should be thin.

Sauté peppers in 3 tablespoons hot oil for 2 minutes. Remove from pan and set aside. Add 3 tablespoons more oil and sauté mushrooms in this oil for 1–2 minutes in high heat so that they will color. Remove mushrooms and set aside. Turn off heat under oil and add garlic and coarsely sliced tomatoes; toss about 30 seconds (you may need to add a bit more oil to pan).

Divide onions among the 3 circles of dough. Spread marinara sauce over onions, then sprinkle on peppers and mushrooms, and next add tomatoes and garlic. Sprinkle all with herbs, seeds, crushed peppers, and crushed seeds. Place each pan (or 2 if they fit) on a cookie sheet and bake 20 minutes on lowest shelf in oven.

Brush visible crust with oil and continue baking 5–10 minutes or until crust is golden brown (or darker if you prefer).

Notes: If you cannot find cake yeast, you can substitute a small package of dry yeast.

If you need a thick marinara sauce, reduce your sauce over medium heat until it thickens.

Herbs and seeds can be crushed with mortar and pestle or with a heavy skillet or wine bottle on a wooden board.

"Peppercorn"

---

4 green bell peppers
2–3 large leeks, carefully
    cleaned
2 Tbs. corn oil
4 red bell peppers
4 ears of corn, with kernels cut
    from cob

2–3 green chili peppers
    (*optional*)
Chopped garlic, desired
    amount

Dice peppers. Slice leeks on the diagonal.

In a large wok* stir-fry† all ingredients, except garlic, in hot corn oil. Toss in chopped garlic, stir a moment, and serve immediately.

YIELD: 2 servings.

* If your stove will not accommodate a large wok, use a small wok or sauté pan. However, since too much in too small a pan will steam, not stir-fry, you may want to stir-fry the peppers first, then the remainder of the vegetables, adding oil a bit at a time, as you need it.

† To stir-fry, heat the oil to hot (a drop of water will splatter and sizzle when dropped into hot oil) and toss vegetables quickly, keeping them moving. In this recipe, the stir-frying should take no longer than 4 minutes, provided you like crunchy vegetables.

Vegetable Fried Rice

2–3 leeks cut on diagonal, white part only

10 fresh mushrooms and/or 8 shitake mushrooms, soaked

12–16 asparagus spears, cut on diagonal

10 snow peas (Chinese pea pods), cleaned

1 cup brown rice

3–4 Tbs. sesame oil

1–2 cloves garlic, minced

7–8 gratings ginger

Dice vegetables into small pieces. Asparagus spears can either be left in longer pieces on diagonal or cut into small diagonals.

Cook rice in 2 cups water, brought to the boil, then turned to a low simmer, covered, for about 40–45 minutes.

Heat 1–2 tablespoons oil in wok or skillet till hot enough for drop of water to sizzle. Stir-fry vegetables quickly, turning and moving them for 1–2 minutes, or until they are done the way you like them. Cooking time will, of course, depend on how large or small you have diced them.

Toss in garlic and ginger, and add rice, turning quickly and adding more oil if needed. Cook only long enough to make certain rice is hot (2 minutes). Serve immediately.

YIELD: 2 servings.

Chinese Stir-Fry Vegetables

24 asparagus spears
4–5 leeks, well cleaned, white
    part only
30 snow peas (Chinese pea
    pods)

1 tsp. sesame oil
1–2 cloves garlic, minced
7–8 gratings ginger

Cut asparagus spears on the diagonal. Cut leeks on the diagonal. Remove stems from snow peas.

Sauté or stir-fry vegetables for about 5 minutes in hot oil. Toss in garlic and ginger,* stir a moment. Serve immediately.

YIELD: 2 servings.

VARIATION 1   Try this dish with broccoli, mushrooms (fresh or shitake mushrooms that have been soaked in warm water and stems removed), leeks, and pea pods.

VARIATION 2   Adding cooked oriental noodles to your stir-fry, or stir-fry mostly cooked noodles and add dry red pepper flakes and a few of the above-mentioned vegetables that have been stir-fried first. Bok choy is good in this recipe; and celery is always a reliable choice.

* Garlic and ginger may be stir-fried first. This is the traditional method, but garlic will be bitter. Also, if you want the leeks to be more well done, cook them 3 minutes alone to start.

Tempura Mazel

Tempura is a Japanese dish. Tidbits are dipped in a batter of flour, water, and egg yolk, sizzled to golden in hot fat (by all means, use your wok for this if you have one), drained, and artistically arranged and served, usually on a doily-lined flat basket. The consistency of the batter (which must be neither too thick nor too thin) and the temperature of the oil (350° is just right) are of the utmost importance. Tempura cannot wait; it must go directly from wok to table.

5 asparagus, cut into 2 or 3 long diagonal pieces

1–2 large carrots, sliced 1/4″ thick on diagonal

10 green beans, ends trimmed

2 small zucchini, cut into thick sticks

1 bell pepper, cut into strips, pith and seeds removed

6 shitake mushrooms, soaked in warm water

6 large parsley sprigs, stems removed, dried

4 Nori seaweed, cut into quarters (available in Japanese markets)

Clean and cut vegetables; make certain they are dry.

Batter:

Ice water

2 1/4 cups flour

3 egg yolks

1 1/2 quarts safflower oil (more if using sauté pan)

Gradually add ice water to flour with a whisk till mixture is the consistency of heavy cream. Beat yolks and whisk into mixture.

Heat oil to 350° in wok or large sauté pan. Dip vegetables into batter and fry till golden (1–2 minutes). Do not crowd pan. Drain.

Chilis Mazel

---

6 fresh green chilis
1 recipe Mazel Cheese Mexican
   (p. 178), warmed
Ice water
¾ cup flour

1 egg yolk
Safflower oil to deep fry (about
   1½ qts.)
1 recipe of cooked Salsa Mazel
   (p. 181)

Slit chilis lengthwise, just long enough to stuff with Mazel Cheese Mexican. Clean out seeds, etc. Stuff with Mazel Cheese mixture and set aside.

Gently whisk enough ice water into flour to make it about the consistency of heavy cream. Beat yolk with a fork, then whisk into batter.

Heat oil to 350°. Dip each chili into batter. Cook in oil till golden (1–2 minutes).* Drain on paper towels.

Served cooked salsa over chilis.

YIELD: 2 servings.

* The timing on deep frying is difficult to pinpoint. Variables include size of pan, the amount of oil used, temperature of oil, desired color of finished product, etc. Do not crowd pan.

Mazel Mex

2½ cups cold water
1¼ cups cornmeal
Generous dash cayenne pepper
    and/or cinnamon
2–3 Tbs. corn oil
3 onions, peeled and coarsely
    chopped
8 large tomatoes, coarsely
    chopped*

1–2 fresh green or jalepeño
    chilis, peeled and coarsely
    chopped
1–2 cloves garlic, peeled and
    minced
1 Tbs. fresh cilantro, chopped
    and torn into leaves
1 Tbs. fresh parsley, chopped

Combine water, cornmeal, and cayenne. Cook, stirring frequently, over medium heat for 5–8 minutes. Pat evenly onto bottom of 8″ x 12″ casserole.

Sauté onions in corn oil until translucent and fairly soft (10–15 minutes). Add tomatoes, chilis, and garlic, and cook 2–3 minutes. Pour mixture over cornmeal base and bake in 350° oven for 20–25 minutes. To serve, sprinkle with cilantro and parsley.

YIELD: 2 servings.

* Although taste is bitter if tomatoes are unpeeled, the peels are an important aid to digestion.

Mazel Enchiladas

6–8 corn tortillas
¼ cup corn oil
2 recipes Mazel Cheese
  Mexican*

1 recipe cooked Salsa Mazel
  (*p. 181*)
1 recipe fresh Salsa Mazel
  (*p. 181*)

Dip corn tortillas in hot corn oil, then into cooked salsa. Fill with Mazel Cheese Mexican, and roll into enchiladas. Cover with cooked salsa. Bake at 350° for 15–20 minutes. Serve with fresh salsa.

VARIATION 1 Add 1 bunch fresh spinach, cooked and chopped, to Mazel Cheese Mexican.

VARIATION 2 Add 1 tablespoon fresh mixed chives and parsley to Mazel Cheese Mexican.

VARIATION 3 Use 1 recipe Mazel Cheese and 1½–2 cups sour cream rather than 2 recipes Mazel Cheese.

YIELD: 2 servings.

* Depending on size of tortillas and how you fill them, you may wind up with a bit of extra filling. If so, add it to the casserole or reserve it for another use. But better too much than too little.

Fried Matzo Mazel

---

3 onions, sliced or chopped
½ stick unsalted butter
6 sheets unsalted matzo,
  soaked in water and
  squeezed

Sauté onions in butter until they are brown and crispy. Add matzo and cook till golden.

YIELD: 2 servings.

Guru 2

Lettuce, Tomato, and Onion on a Toasted Buttered Bagel

BREAD

Bagels

---

1 pkg. yeast	½ cup whole wheat flour
1½ cups warm water	1 Tbs. bran
4 cups unbleached flour	6 qts. boiling water

Dissolve yeast in ½ cup of the water. Cover, put in a warm place, and let set 15 minutes. Add yeast mixture and the remaining cup of water to flour/bran mixture to make a soft dough. Knead for 5 minutes on floured board. Cover dough and let rise 15 minutes. Punch dough down, divide into 8-10 pieces and rolling them, join ends of each together to form a circle. Cover and let rise another 20 minutes. Drop bagels into boiling water for one minute. Transfer to ungreased nonstick cookie sheet. Bake in 350° oven for 30 minutes till brown.

VARIATION   Sauté ¼ cup chopped onion in unsalted butter and sprinkle on bagels before baking.

IX

Parties and Other Falderal:
The Conscious Combiner
Goes Social

Two things fatten people up—their social life and their emotional life. I fall prey to both. Many of you do, too. Unfortunately, we are members of a food-oriented society. Business meetings take place over breakfast, lunch, cocktails, and dinner. We entertain with food. We socialize with food. We celebrate with food. Now, with the rash of gourmet-cooking classes, we're learning with food, too. One-upmanship these days seems to ride on outcooking one another. Cooking and eating are our number-one national pastime.

I'd be a fool to ask you to give all that up—I'm certainly not willing to, and I haven't. Obviously, in the first weeks of any diet, you will have to make *some* social adjustments. Such is the case on any weight-loss regimen. But eventually, you can schedule your eating orgies to fully take advantage of your social calendar—with permission, without guilt, and with pleasure.

In the Beginning

Above all, don't make any social sacrifices while you are on the Beverly Hills Diet. It is important to experience food in your real world from the very beginning, to make conscious food choices in your natural environment from the very beginning.

203

Don't build a sterile artifice around you and the Beverly Hills Diet. Remember, diet means way of life, and social integration is a key part of my methodology. After all, do you think the Beverly Hills' elite live in a vacuum?

Don't use your social life as an excuse. One actress went to a formal dinner party, and course by course, she ate her figs. Horsewoman and businesswoman Jackie Applebaum goes to dinner parties about six nights a week. She calls her hostess in advance, explains her diet, and finds out if any of the menu meshes with her needs. If not, Jackie brings her own food and has it served appropriately.

"I have found it's far better to alert my hostess ahead of time than to pick at my food and make her squirm and wonder if something is wrong with her cooking," explains Jackie.

Dick Martin took his strawberries onto the golf course, his watermelon to the studio, and his grapes to a dinner party.

Make a commitment before you go to a party. If you are on a grape day, eat grapes, and that's it. Remember, nobody can *make* you taste anything. There will be more dinners and more parties. Your social life will go on and on. What are a few weeks out of an entire lifetime? Especially when you are in the process of creating an eternal skinny?

Take your food with you, or ask your hostess to provide it for you. Otherwise, you'll become a victim and/or a martyr.

Don't be ashamed to admit you're on a diet. If you are conspicuously fat and you are eating what the other guests are eating, they are probably wondering why you're *not* on a diet. If you're approaching skinny and dieting because you want to shed those final ten, or if you're maintaining and want the extra energy, you can get away with anything.

One of the best "social" excuses I have heard was from a woman from New York who was most anxious to go on my diet because so many of her friends had been successful. But she kept breaking appointments. Her problem? "I can't go on your diet," she finally confessed. "I date." "Oh," I responded, "and your dates don't notice that you're fat?"

As a Combiner

If it is a choice between gaining weight or not, your life becomes more complicated. You can always choose to miscombine or do an Open Human. Sometimes it will be worth it and other times it won't.

I'm going to concentrate on eating socially to *maintain* or *lose weight*. After all, that's what Conscious Combining is all about. We all know how to gain weight. What I want to teach you is how to make the right choices to get and stay thin and still be socially acceptable, because just how socially acceptable are fat people, especially to themselves.

Once you have succeeded on the first few weeks of the Beverly Hills Diet, your food choices at parties open up. When making choices, you can always go Open Human. If you think about food when it doesn't count, you don't have to think about it when it does.

When I go to a party, I have one thought in mind as food passes before me. Is it worth it? I know that for every bite of food that goes into my mouth, something else can't.

If you want to drink wine and be assured of losing weight, go on an Open Fruit day. That means that at the party, you will eat fruit and drink wine. Cheese and fruit have become highly fashionable, so fruit shouldn't be a problem, even if you don't bring your own. Skip the cheese, of course.

On a Resnick Open you can drink your choice of liquors. It also means, you will recall, no eating and setting yourself up for it properly by eating fruit only, if you want to drink wine. If you have had carbs, you can have any of the carb alcohols but no wine. If you have eaten protein, you cannot do a Resnick Open.

On Open Carb, you can drink any of the grain alcohols like scotch, bourbon, and vodka and eat any of the carbs—the crudités, the chips, and the crackers.

If you are eating and not drinking and really want to lose, forego miscombination. Pick out just the protein hors d'oeuvres (meatballs are one of my favorites) or just the carbs. You'll need to do some experimenting to learn just what your body will tolerate in terms of salt and other spoilers, etc. Remember, the physical laws are constant. Individuals are not.

If you taste something and it isn't good, spit it out—surreptitiously.

Avoid very salty foods. Try to resist the overloaded chips and nuts.

Avoid gelatin molds, cheese, pretzels, and dips.

Plan for the party. Set yourself up enzymatically, so you can make your choice on the spot and go either protein or carb. Avoid being locked into what you must eat. Don't begin the day of a party with protein. Stay "enzymatically open."

Quiche is a treacherous miscombination. Make sure it's worth it. There are some pretty bad quiches on the cocktail-party circuit.

Be aware of nibbling to fill social gaps and those moments of insecurity. When you think about it, do you go to a cocktail party to eat or socialize? Try concentrating on the conversation instead of the eating. You know that as soon as you put something in your mouth, someone will invariably ask you a question.

Don't station yourself next to the pastry table. Try standing away from the goodies. It helps a lot.

"Getting high" pulverizes our will power and turns some of us into raving food maniacs. Don't use it as an excuse.

Before one morsel passes those lips, check everything out, including the desserts. That way you'll know exactly what you will want to do—Open Carb, Open Protein, Resnick Open, Open

Dessert, etc. Whatever your choice, forget the regret and stick to it.

On the other hand, just because it's there, you are under no obligation to eat it.

I always carry something with me for security, just in case there is nothing I really want. My cache of cashews, for example. Often I'll reject everything at a cocktail party in favor of those cashews.

If you are caught at a party where the food is not only not worth eating, but certainly not worth gaining for—something you don't even like to begin with, and you know you'll leave ravenous, and if it will end within say an hour and a half, think instead of something wonderful and legal you will eat the moment you escape and fake eating. No one will notice.

Once, when I was playing this role to the hilt, I suggested I might venture forth for *more* moussaka after lumping my first serving untouched in a small pile off-center on my plate. My outspoken dinner partner's response? "You ate enough. You don't need anymore." I stopped on my way home for my favorite cheesecake.

Don't let the particular situation or place dictate what you eat. Make your own choices. Stay in control. Please yourself, not someone else. You'll end up pleasing the rest of the world, too.

Don't revert to old habits.

For the first time in his life, Greg had just achieved slimhood. We were at a cocktail party, and he was nibbling chips and pretzels. He, of course, can eat whatever he chooses. He's skinny. But it looked to me like unconscious munching. I asked him what he had eaten that day. Chicken, he said. The buffet table was bursting with an abundance of protein—steak tartare, rare roast beef, turkey, cheese, even a fabulous cheesecake! Greg could have eaten almost anything there and still maintained or even lost weight. But he blew it by breaking the protein rule—on something that wasn't even worth it, that he wasn't even aware of or experiencing. A case of old habits. . . .

There are times when you clearly compromise. So concede with dignity. After all, tomorrow is another day.

There we were, Susie and I, at the home of a friend who was touted to be a chef of great skill. It was just the three of us. The meal was a disaster. The tempura batter slid off the vegetables, the oil was tepid, the vegetables soggy. It was magnificently presented. Our host thought it was wonderful. We couldn't fake it. We gave up and ate. Well, it was just one meal. . . . We knew pineapple would be our salvation.

Holidays

Traditionally, holidays have always represented an opportunity to go crazy—those special occasions when all of our excuses are allowed, when everybody is blowing it. No one is watching. But that's the old diet consciousness that says holidays are the last supper.

There is no need for you, as a Conscious Combiner, to eat yourself *under* the table, because there's nothing on that table that you can't have tomorrow.

Think of holidays as a testing ground for your new consciousness. This is *the* time to let your skinny voice shout.

Last Easter, one of my clients, a society hostess of impressive repute, had her staff serve her watermelon cut in the shapes of crosses, Easter eggs, and bunnies. She had more fun than anyone!

Skinny people don't get crazy just because it's Thanksgiving. They know when enough is enough. So do you.

If, on a holiday, you decide to go Open Human, fine. Lots of Conscious Combiners do. Remember, though, to eat with one hand, one bite at a time, watching and emulating a skinny person. It's not how much you can get in how short a time, but how long you can make the pleasure last. Remember that if you don't eat it all today, it will still be here tomorrow. It won't leave the planet.

Give yourself permission to enjoy the holiday without guilt. Next Thanksgiving, give yourself something to be thankful for —the body you have dreamed of and the methodology and the skinny voice to keep it.

You can choose simply to maintain your present weight. Or you can decide to happily eat your way through the holidays while losing. Since holidays spawn so many leftovers, you can probably get it all in—over several days, anyway. Another way of making the pleasure last and last and last: Go Open Carb one day, Open Protein the next, and Open dessert the third.

Perhaps, because they are so aware, and because holidays are no longer an excuse, my clients rarely gain much weight over the holidays. Let me share a sample menu that many of us followed last Thanksgiving. Use your imagination, and use it as a yardstick for other holiday menus.

Thanksgiving

WITHOUT GUILT, GOING HUNGRY, GIVING UP, OR
GAINING WEIGHT

Choice of Turkey or Stuffing

or

Potatoes, Sweet, Yams, any style (candied or otherwise)

1 Dessert (optional)

or

3 Desserts

or

Open Miscombination
Examples:
Turkey and Stuffing
Turkey and Candied Yams
Turkey and Pumpkin Pie

or

Open Human

Pick any of the combinations, and eat as much as you want. Once you have made your decision, that is it. No "just one bite." That doesn't belong. Eat until you are really full, until you have had enough. Not included in your choices are string beans and salad. You can have them 364 days of the year. Why bother on Thanksgiving? If you decide on an Open Miscombination or Open Human, follow through with care and discipline.

Eat your Open Human the way Laurie did. "Thanksgiving on a diet meant being able to eat whatever I wanted, from Mom's apple pie to Aunt Elana's stuffing. For once in my life, I was able to really taste what I was eating. I think I probably could have told you the spices each contained. Eating just a little bit of everything felt so much better. After dinner was over, I felt so good because, even though I had eaten until I was full, I knew that I hadn't blown it. And getting on the scale this morning and seeing that I hadn't gained any weight made yesterday even better."

Birthdays

Birthdays are really let-loose days because it's your day and nobody else's. Even those who harp about our fat will take us out, pile it high, and egg us on. Well, this year, you have something to celebrate—being a "born-again skinny."

To reinforce my own life choice of being a skinny, because that 170-pound whale that I once was is always lurking, I choose to make my birthday one of the most austere days of my year. Almost like a day of worship and reverence for myself, my health, and my skinny being.

Too well I know that what once was can always be again. Those lusting little fat cells are poised at attention, waiting eagerly for their chance to plump up again. Instead of eating I buy myself a present—something special that I have looked forward to during the year.

Of course, many of my clients ignore my example and celebrate with food, and that's okay because they immediately turn to the recoups and recover. Ask Jackie Applebaum, who on her birthday not only sampled seven entrees at The Bistro Garden, but also had three scoops of pralines-and-cream ice cream for dessert. Within three days of her birthday she weighed a pound less than she had before she began the celebration. Don't use holidays as an excuse. You don't need one anymore. . . .

Weddings, Banquets, and Their Ilk

These deserve a separate category because they have one thing in common—the food is prepared en masse. Before you make your decision about which way to go, think about whether you really want to blow it on a meal prepared for hundreds. Is this *really* the time to do an Open Human?

Since there's always a salad and bread and butter, Open Carb is usually the best choice. The protein is either wading in sauce or drenched in salt.

It's easy for most public facilities to be accommodating. That, after all, is their business. Call the catering department ahead of time and ask for a special meal. You'll almost always be able to get baked potatoes or a vegetable plate and, yes, even fruit. Remember Barbara, the wife of the councilman? She lost forty-five pounds on the banquet circuit by using this system.

The size of a wedding party will sometimes dictate your decision. If it's small and intimate, with good food, your choice will be tougher. As with the rest of the world, there are always exceptions. But generally, mass affairs are not worth blowing it on.

X

Garçon! Caviar, Please

RESTAURANTS AND OTHER SNEAKY PLACES

Go. I don't expect you to become a hermit. Au contraire! You don't think we sit home in Beverly Hills, do you? But when you do go to a restaurant, any restaurant, remember that you are paying for much more than the food; you are paying for the service. The staff is there to accommodate you, not vice versa. No matter what you want, don't be afraid to ask for it. You'll always encounter that rare surly waiter. But that's his problem. Be assertive.

For Weight Loss

When you're on pineapple, you're on pineapple. Period. Not a whole lot of choice there. Soon you'll be able to eat, and eat well, at your favorite restaurant. But while you're on the strict weight-loss segment of the Beverly Hills Diet, before you have become a Conscious Combiner, you simply won't have a choice.

There might even be times, after you're on maintenance, when you're already committed to a certain kind of day, and a last-minute invitation comes along that isn't worth gaining for.

Remember that your life is filled with last-minute invitations, some better than others.

I've been to some of the most splendid restaurants in the world and have just eaten pineapple or berries or baked potato or salad or bread and butter. I know those restaurants are not leaving the planet. They aren't burning down. They'll be there tomorrow.

Going to a restaurant is not a license to blow it. Count the number of times in an average week you are in one. Count everything—every time you're out of the house for food. Write it down. If you make an exception for each of those occasions, if you give in to all of them, there is only one thing that will leave the planet: your newfound hipbones!

How many restaurants are really worth blowing it for? Look at your list. Mark those that are, and schedule them in.

But back to the scheduled diet days. There are lots of ways to handle a watermelon day at a restaurant. Call in advance and ask the maitre d' if he has what you need. If he can't provide it, ask him if he will serve you your own food if you bring it with you. If you can't call in advance, take your food with you, and speak to the maitre d' upon arriving. Tell him you are on a special diet, that this is all you can eat, and would they please serve it to you.

Of course, offer to pay a service charge—whatever a normal meal would have cost. After all, it is presumptuous of us to think we can monopolize a place in a restaurant without paying. It is, after all, the way they make their money. Despite this fact, you probably won't be charged.

If it's a coffee shop and there's no maitre d', tell the waitress what you're up to, and offer to pay. Always be prepared with your food. Remember, don't be a victim or a martyr.

My new clients find that one of the hardest parts of the

Beverly Hills Diet is confronting restaurant personnel—but only in the beginning: Believe me, *it's easy*, it's fun, eventually it becomes a game. Don't let restaurants spell your demise.

One young client of mine went on a blind date with another couple to a Mexican restaurant and had the waitress serve her the watermelon she had brought along. "It was delicious. Maybe it wasn't enchiladas, but it was still good watermelon. I looked at my friends' food, and it looked really good to me. But knowing I would lose at least a pound by eating watermelon, there was no way I would have even tasted theirs. I knew if I did, I would get on the scale in the morning and feel angry, guilty, and depressed—and for what, a taste of an enchilada? The next day, I weighed one pound less, and I felt terrific."

Don't go to a restaurant empty-handed because you don't want to "impose" or draw attention to yourself. Don't just sit there drinking black coffee shrouded in martyrdom while everyone around you indulges. You'll be miserable, and those around you may be uncomfortable. Don't use what you perceive as other people's discomfort at your eating grapes as an excuse to order something else.

As long as you are eating something, most people relax. And don't keep your food hidden away and furtively sneak it out bite by bite. There is nothing to be ashamed of.

Susan Haymer, a highly successful businesswoman, had real difficulty stating her case for her different manner of eating for two reasons: 1) she was thin enough so people didn't consider her fat, and 2) she was afraid she would forfeit her prime tables at her favorite restaurants by Conscious Combining eating. Finally, confronted by a seemingly insurmountable plateau, and upon my insistence, she ordered triple raspberries at a business luncheon. Not only did she not suffer so much as an iota of disdain at the chic French restaurant Ma Maison, the next morning she was down 2¾ pounds! Susan had welcomed Conscious Combining into *all* phases of her life, and in so doing, she conquered her mind/body split and ended her plateau.

Sam Brown, a regular at the sleek Beverly Hills restaurant Mateos, found himself on a popcorn night having promised to take his best girl to his favorite Italian restaurant for her birthday dinner. Sam walked in with a brown paper bag filled with popcorn and asked the maitre d', "Have you got popcorn on the menu tonight, Matty?" Matty cheerfully accommodated Sam with a bowl.

It gets easier each and every time, and you will begin having fun with it. There may even come a day when you *choose* to eat raisins instead of anything on the menu because that's what you *really* want.

If salt is not a major problem for you, if you aren't a big bloater, don't make a big deal out of it. If you are, you'll pick and choose the times you get "salted." Ask the waiter *not* to use salt. That may or may not work. You may have to resort to more extreme measures, such as threatening to put the paramedics on standby if the cook so much as thinks about salt while preparing your meal.

Beware of hidden sugar and salt in salad dressing. The house vinaigrette almost always has salt or sugar or both. Same for sauces.

French restaurants are good choices because they have good fruit, especially berries. Order a double or triple serving. Mark Rosenberg, a movie-studio executive, lost fifty pounds, and never once did eating pineapple for breakfast or grapes for lunch interfere with his daily business breakfasts and lunches.

When you are on a Mono Meal, you will probably eat much more slowly than those around you, so be sure to order your food to begin with the first course, no matter what it is. You can always order more.

Don't, I repeat, don't sit around and feel sorry for yourself. You have permission to order seconds or thirds. You can eat as much as you want. You're getting skinny; what is there to feel sorry about?

Still Losing, But Combining

When you look at the menu, use your imagination. Just because it says appetizer or main course or salad, it doesn't have to be served in that order.

Your one objective is to eat when everyone else is eating. A psychiatrist client found herself at the Blue Fox in San Francisco for dinner, and she was on an Open Protein night. She had cracked crab as an appetizer, baked white fish as her main course, and for dessert her date had chocolate mousse while she had scampi!

On a potato night in Los Angeles, I had the waiter serve a baked potato to me for each course. What I didn't finish, he swept away only to return with a new one each time the rest of my party was served a new course. He served me four potatoes.

Remember your best bet for weight loss is the Mono Meal. Second best weight-losing choice is Open Carb or Open Protein. Needless to say, Open Human or Open Miscombination meals are no guarantee that you will lose or even maintain.

French Restaurants

A veritable garden of exquisitely prepared greens!

Open Carb should be no problem in a French restaurant. There are always marvelous salads. My favorite is spinach, watercress, endive, and mushrooms.

For salad dressing, it's safest to order unmixed oil and vinegar with fresh seasonings on the side. There's likely to be salt and sugar in the premixed. I often take my own dressing in a purse-size bottle (the ones liquid garlic come in).

The bread is always fabulous, and all French restaurants have unsalted butter. They use it extensively in their cooking. You can also count on a large assortment of fresh vegetables, which can be cooked to your taste. The Bjorg Special—salad, bread and butter, and a dessert, usually a chocolate soufflé—was spawned by a French-restaurant habitué who loved carbohydrates more than protein.

Potatoes are not the best choice in a French restaurant because they're usually drenched in butter or a cream sauce.

If you choose Open Carb, remember not to confine yourself to stereotyped orders. Juggle the menu items to suit your whims. Ask them to do something special. French cooks are famous for their creativity, and they love a challenge.

For Open Protein, veal chops, beef, fish, and seafood are all wonderful.

Beware of the Frenchman's sauces. Because of their high salt and/or sugar content, they can be the nemesis of the Conscious Combiner.

Italian Restaurants

Unfortunately, the problem is the cheese. There is no place for cheese on your diet while you are losing weight. Once you're on maintenance, however, you can carefully reintegrate it. Remember to eat cheese only as the last meal of the day, because once cheese passes your lips you are inhibiting the digestibility of anything else you eat after it.

Open Carb. Italian restaurants are Open Carbers' playgrounds. To refresh your memory, Open Carb is any three carbs, only two of which can be maxi carbs. You can have three pastas though, because they represent a *single* maxi-carb type.

Pasta can be prepared in a splendid variety of ways without proteins—for example, aglio e olio (garlic and olive oil), al burro (butter and garlic), and with a variety of vegetables, such as broccoli, mushrooms, and asparagus. The options are endless. Why not try three different noodles with three different sauces? One of my own P-W-P (pasta with pleasure) nights was as follows:

APPETIZER
Fettucine al burro

MAIN COURSE
Vermicelli aglio e olio, fresh parsley, and mushrooms

DESSERT
Spaghetti with marinara sauce

I ate it all and didn't gain an ounce.

If you want a little variety in your meal, how about a salad sans garbanzo beans, cheese, and salami? Eggplant sautéed in olive oil with fresh garlic and mushrooms is fabulous. Or try zucchini and eggplant dipped in flour and deep-fried.

The bread, of course, is spectacular. Make sure the butter is unsalted.

Desserts generally aren't worth it. Most contain protein, so unless you are on an Open Dessert night or an Open Miscombination or an Open Human, you can't have them.

Open Protein. Italian restaurants are known for excellent veal, and osso bucco is my favorite. Fish and chicken are usually great, too. As at French restaurants, there's a plethora of choices. Just watch out for the sauces and the cheese. Remember, sauces are carbs, and they don't mesh with protein.

Oriental Restaurants

The worst part of an oriental meal is the MSG (monosodium glutamate). It causes some people to experience what is known as the Chinese restaurant syndrome—that empty feeling after a Chinese meal, a nagging headache, and a large percent of the bloating that follows your meal. Designed to perk up your taste buds, it can also muddle your brain and confound your nervous system. It reacts negatively against your chemical balance.

Try asking your waiter to leave out the MSG. Maybe he will. One way to tell for sure is to wait five minutes after taking your first bite. If it contains MSG and you are sensitive to it, you will feel a tingling on the tips of your fingers and the back of your neck. There is good news, however. Some of the newer and almost all of the better Chinese restaurants have stopped using MSG because there's been such a public outcry against it.

The second killer in a Chinese restaurant is the sodium-laden soy sauce. An integral part of Chinese food, it's hard to avoid. I, your basic bloater, avoid it. This is a choice you'll have to make for yourself. Because there is a recoup and because Conscious Combining is never a never. If you decide to go straight without MSG and soy sauce, then ask to have your food cooked with lots of garlic and ginger. It's marvelous!

Open Carb. Vegetables and stir-fried rice is one of my favorites. (Hold the egg please; it adds consistency and protein, making it a miscom, but no flavor.) Noodles, you know, originated in China, and Chinese restaurants do wonderful things with them. Chow mein and all its many variations are delicious too. Just make sure there's no protein, salt, or soy sauce included in any of the carb dishes. Be careful with soups. They're probably made with chicken stock and thus self-defeating.

Open Protein. Most protein dishes can be adapted for Conscious Combiners. If vegetables are mixed in, just push them aside. The presence of vegetables, you'll recall, doesn't make the protein indigestible. It's the protein that dramatically interferes with the digestion of the carbs. Watch the sauces.

Japanese Restaurants

Japanese food is tricky, too, because of the soy sauce and the MSG. Your Open Carb choices are far more limited than with Chinese food. Vegetable tempura is a great exception. If they leave out the egg in the batter. Obviously, rice is a mainstay. Also the stir-fried and steamed vegetables—sans protein.

Your best bet in a Japanese restaurant is Open Protein. I adore Sashimi (raw fish). Kobe beef or any of their mixed dishes can be adapted. Lots of Combiners bring along their Mazel Dressing to use as a dip. It's much better than the house sauces and far less destructive.

Remember that the base of Japanese sauces is soy sauce, and if you're a bloater that will translate into pounds tomorrow. Always ask yourself "Is it worth it?" and if the answer is yes, then go ahead and enjoy it because tomorrow is another day and it's here for you to enjoy because you have the tools for eternal slimhood.

Mexican Restaurants

Cheese breathes life into a Mexican restaurant. Beware! Despite this, Mexican restaurants are easier to handle than you might at first think.

Open Carb. Try chips and salsa. You'd be surprised how few Mexican restaurants salt their chips. Check it out. Watch for sugar in the salsa. A tostado salad minus the protein; the beans, cheese, and avocado are great. Try flour tortillas or corn tortillas with unsalted butter. If you can, talk your waiter into producing a cheeseless enchilada filled with onions and sour cream; that's a carb and fat combo, perfectly acceptable and delicious to boot. Add some salsa, and you'll think you're in Acapulco.

Open Protein. Carne asada is excellent. So is fish. Or if you're an avocado lover, you're in luck: it is a mainstay of Mexican restaurants. Guacamole is a miscombination, however.

A Wholesome American Restaurant

Open Carb. Now it gets really easy. American restaurants always have a variety of vegetables, potatoes, bread, salads, and desserts.

Open Protein. A big choice of unadulterated meats, fowl, and fish. Just make sure you eat right along with everyone else, and if you want three different items, you might want to select all of them or two of them from among the entrees.

We must not make restaurants a big problem. They aren't. They are much easier than parties or banquets. Nothing will appear on your plate to tempt you that you didn't specifically order. Your selection is immense. I have yet to find a restaurant that didn't offer Combiners a happy choice. Plus, restaurants exist to serve you, the customer. They are there to cater to your food needs. If you're gracious and explain what you're doing, you'll convert even the most snarly waiter.

Restaurants will always be a part of your life. Now is the time to put them into perspective. Don't let them interfere with your skinniness. It's so unnecessary. It's so self-defeating.

One of the biggest difficulties is deciding which way to go—Open Carb or Open Protein. Remind yourself that nothing is leaving the planet. This isn't a last-supper decision. The restaurant is not burning down. If the choice is that tough, go back tomorrow, and eat what you are passing up today. You're not going to be hungry. You're not going to be deprived. You're not going to be bored. Compare the Beverly Hills Diet to any other diet you've ever endured, and you'll celebrate.

Alan and Jack, two of my clients, ate at The Palm at least twice a week. Yet every time Jack went, he crammed it all in—potatoes, onions, bread and butter, steak, lobster, and cheesecake. I couldn't make him acknowledge that The Palm was a regular part of his life. In the six weeks he came to see me, he went there fourteen times. Each time he had to have it all. Obviously, he had suppressed his skinny voice. Alan, on the other hand, ate potatoes and onions one time, steak and lobster another. Not only did he not feel deprived or go hungry, but he developed a new body in the process—one that was twenty-seven pounds lighter. Need I add, Jack was not one of my success stories.

If you let that skinny voice take over, eating out can be a joy—untained by the guilt that comes from gorging.

Another client tells of his first trip to New York City as a Combiner. He ate at his favorite restaurant, a restaurant that had always epitomized the ultimate in dining to him. "I enjoyed ordering my meal and finishing it, and—for the first time in my life—stopping when I was full," he said. "After all that time, all those meals of shoveling it in, I realized *inside* that it wasn't leaving the planet. I could go there again tomorrow. It was the first time it had ever happened. And then to go home and find I hadn't gained one ounce!"

As still another client points out, "I have given myself permission to enjoy eating out. I don't have to go off in a corner and eat anymore. I can now eat openly. I used to get only half the enjoyment I now get out of a restaurant."

Restaurants are a regular part of your life. You don't have to eat everything each time you go. They will not all burn down. And they are there to serve *you*. Plus, by now, many will be familiar with the Beverly Hills Diet. So spread the word, incorporate restaurants into your eating world, and make me proud of you.

COMBINERS ON THE GO:
TRAVEL AND ITS SPECIAL
PITFALLS

Getting There

Conscious Combiners travel—some often and regularly; others, it's one big trip a year. But make no mistake about it, we do not live in a vacuum. Like restaurants, travel must be integrated into your Beverly Hills Diet. It must not be used as an excuse to make exceptions in your choice of foods. Just as restaurants are a constant in your life, so is travel. Never forget that the Beverly Hills Diet is a way of life to be integrated into every aspect of your life. And you do eat when you travel, don't you?

For starters, take a scale with you; remember what happened to me in New York (see page 129). There are many lightweight, inexpensive bathroom scales that won't take up any more room in your suitcase than a handbag.

If you're driving, it's easy: just take your food with you. Usually the restaurants at your destination are far superior to those en route. But if there are some good ones along the way and you know about them in advance, eat accordingly and plan to schedule them in.

Frankly, I can't understand why anyone going on a vacation or a business trip, much of which invariably revolves around food and eating, would kick it off by eating airplane food. What a waste! No matter how you travel—first class, coach or economy, airline food is all the same: precooked, microwaved, oversalted, and heaven knows what else. And who knows how long it's been sitting around! As a Combiner, would you consciously choose to eat a TV dinner? Why waste an Open Human on airline food?

But, if you insist, the best of all possible choices would be to eat only protein, or special-order your meal when you make your reservation. Some airlines will even accommodate you with a pineapple, strawberry, or even a papaya plate. If they won't, choose vegetarian (be sure to tell them *no cheese*), seafood, or low-sodium plates. They cost nothing extra and the airlines provide these special meals as a matter of course.

Instead of eating airline food, many Combiners choose to bring their own with them. You probably will too. The fact that Sandy and Bob Steiner were on the Concorde didn't stop them from taking along their strawberries to accompany the champagne they were served.

An ABC executive, Philip Blumberg, takes a whole watermelon on his transcontinental flights and asks the steward(ess) to cut it on board. For someone else, it's bagels. The time of day, the length of the flight, and what you plan to do when you arrive at your destination will determine what type of food you bring with you. In the daytime, I usually take strawberries or dried fruit. The dried fruit's convenient because you can stow any leftovers for later on in your trip. If it's a long flight, and I know I will not be going out to dinner when I arrive, I opt for grapes. This is the first choice of my transcontinental flyers. At night, I usually take nuts. But I've also taken unsalted potato chips, huge bags of popcorn, even cold chicken. For me, airplanes are for nibbling, so why not take advantage of them? I have yet to peer over at my seatmate's tray and not feel infinitely superior in my choice of foods.

Seasoned travelers and Conscious Combiners know that gorging in the air significantly compounds any jet lag you may suffer.

What to Do When You Get There

It all depends on where you're going. Refer back to restaurants (page 213) for guidelines.

By now, fruit has become an integral part of your life. If you're wise, you'll begin at least 80 percent of your days with fruit. After all, what are you giving up? What did you formerly have for breakfast? If you are like most of my clients, it was usually the meal you skipped.

Fruit, as you have learned, is the key to eternal slimhood—the depository of the vital enzymes. Do not skip it. Remember, those enzymes are digesting what you had the day before and setting you up for the day that is ahead. If you do little else in terms of Conscious Combining when you travel other than beginning your day with fruit, you will very likely maintain your weight. Enzymatically, pineapple, papaya, or berries (in that order) should be your first choice. Apples should be next, then the neutrals. And, if all else fails, you can always find grapefruit. While it's obviously not the most desirable choice, it's better than a nonfruit one. Oranges also beat out croissants and café au lait as a choice when pineapple is not available.

The only fruits that aren't an improvement over none at all are the melons. They bloat you. Also, don't forget that grapes and watermelon should be eaten only as all-day fruits, so if you are inclined to eat them just for breakfast—don't.

If you're trying to *lose* weight while on a trip, the more fruit meals, the better. This book was written in Hawaii, surrounded by a bevy of Beverly Hills Dieters on the Kahala Hilton Hotel beach. We all ate to our hearts' content in this magic land of the pineapple and we maintained and loved it.

If fruit for lunch is possible, great; if not, a carb lunch, either Mono or Open is always workable while losing, wherever you happen to be. A lovely salad, vegetables, even pasta!

The FCP (fruit/carb/protein) day is usually safe, easy and fun while traveling. The fewer the miscombinations, the better. But please, don't be afraid to schedule in a few; obviously, you won't gain every time you miscombine, but you are challenging the odds. Do make the miscombinations count. If you miscombine at breakfast or lunch, remember to stick to protein for the rest of the day.

Even a cruise no longer provides a good excuse to cheat. There's so much food, and so much time to eat it and so many opportunities to eat that if you don't eat it all now, there is always later.

Engelbert Humperdinck went on a concert tour that circled the U.S. and wound up in England. While in England, Engelbert, ever-loyal to his native foods, ate Yorkshire pudding one night and roast beef another. He continued to lose weight.

Sally Kellerman went to Israel to shoot a picture on location and, to the disbelief of the crew, happily ate pasta, vegetables, and bread and butter. And Sally lost weight, too.

You can do the same thing. Without sacrifice. Without missing a single taste sensation. Simply spread it out, and make every bite count. Above all, remember that the food is not leaving the planet. Even if the place where you're eating is not one you visit every day, that same meal, that same pastry, that same pizza, will be there the next time—and the next. If it's not? If it's *really* not? Then maybe this is an instance when you should make plans for having it. For example, I wouldn't think of going to Chicago without scheduling in an Uno's pizza.

Like restaurants, travel can serve as an excuse to blow it. But think. Do you want to come home and put all your new clothes in storage? I don't think so, because now you don't really need an excuse anymore. Haven't I taken them all away? What can't you eat? What can't you have?

Travel is a good time to test your skinny voice. If you're on vacation, it may be overly ambitious to expect to stick to a weight-loss Beverly Hills Diet. A watermelon day while skiing in Aspen? A papaya day while touring the pyramids of Egypt?

Don't be foolish; don't set unrealistic goals. That mistake is a carry-over from your old fat consciousness. Use your trip as a time to mend that mind/body split: to acknowledge where you are today; to experience and *feel* where you are today. Why not just maintain? Come home weighing what you did when you left. Isn't that challenge enough? What have you got to lose?

XI

Conscious Combiners
Have All the Answers

The following questions are those most often asked by my clients. When someone asks me a question, they never get just a simple yes or no. I always explain why I am asking them to eat a certain way because I feel it is important to truly understand this lifelong program of eating. I want you to have the answers, too. But, please, refer to the appropriate section of my book for a more complete discussion of any area.

How much will I lose in the first five weeks?

The average weight loss for women is fifteen to twenty pounds. Men, those lucky devils, lose more, usually anywhere from twenty to thirty pounds.

I hate pineapple. What do I do?

The only substitute for pineapple is strawberries, and they're only part strength. The intensely concentrated, special enzymes in pineapple burn up fat. They are the heart of the Beverly Hills Diet. Try pineapple. You'll probably grow to love it. It's the closest thing to a miracle food that exists.

Can I eat just before bedtime?

You can eat any time you want from the time you open your eyes until you close them.

Do I have to eat all eight ounces of the raisins?

Yes, but you don't have to eat them all at once. If you start and stop—fine. Just finish them before you move on to the next food. Specific amounts are spelled out to achieve a very definite nutritional result, and it is important to eat them all.

How much water should I drink?

As much or as little as you want. Because most of the fruit you're eating has such a high percentage of water, you are getting all you need. Unlike a high-protein regimen, the Beverly Hills Diet does not deplete your body of essential fluids and require that you replenish them.

Why can't I have lime on my papaya?

Lemon and lime interact to neutralize the enzymes we're trying to activate—the pepsin in your stomach and the papain in the papaya. Lemon and lime thwart the very chemical action we are trying to trigger.

Won't I lose more if I eat less?

No. First, you stand a good chance of diluting the enzymatic action of whatever it is you're eating. And second, if you eat less, you'll be hungry, which is to be avoided at all costs on the Beverly Hills Diet. Remember, you are losing weight by feeding your body, not by starving it. If you don't eat the food you won't lose.

Won't I feel tired on this program?

On the contrary, you'll probably have more energy than you've ever had in your life. Remember, because the Beverly Hills Diet focuses on high-energy foods and maximizes the energy potential of those foods, it is an exceptionally high-energy way of eating. Most clients find they need far less sleep than they required before. You probably will, too.

Won't J be living in the bathroom after eating all that fruit?

Hopefully, but probably not. Diarrhea is not as common a reaction as you might think. Besides, how else does fat leave your body? It isn't magically absorbed into the cosmos. Remember, the Beverly Hills Diet burns, feeds, and *washes*. Remember, too, the fourth step in the digestive process is elimination.

J have to cook for my family. Can't J at least taste what J'm making?

No. Every bite counts. Believe me. It wasn't the special occasions or the big meals that fattened you up in the first place. It was most likely the unconscious nibbling and tasting that piled up the pounds.

Think of your body as a machine. Turning your ignition key, for example, starts your car's motor regardless of whether you drive for a second or an hour. The same applies to your body's enzymatic system—it is fully activated regardless of whether you eat a single bite or a whole meal.

What if J cheat?

It won't be the first time, and it won't be the last. That's why I developed the corrective counterparts. That's their miracle. Don't beat yourself over the head, or worse, give yourself license to go completely crazy. Check the "corrective counterparts," and do what is necessary to correct any weight gain. Don't exaggerate its importance. Instead, think of all the times you didn't cheat.

Jf sugar is so bad for you, why do you give us all that sugar in the fruit?

It is a totally different kind of sugar. The quantity and quality of what we typically think of as sugar and the glucose that comes from fruit are *vastly* different. Food should do two things:

provide nutrients and energy. Fruit does both. It provides an extremely high calibre of instant energy, and it feeds our body essential minerals and vitamins.

Sugars, like candy, whose end products are sucrose, do provide energy, but they are virtually deficient nutritionally, since they contain no vitamins or minerals. In fact, in their processing by your body, these sugars actually drain your body of critical nutrients.

So why is refined sugar allowed at all?

Good question. Sugar, salt, and additives are among the three worst things we can put in our bodies. But who among us is going to give up something we love—forever? Even if we know it is bad for us?

The problem with most diets is there are too many nevers. Just knowing that we have to give up something forever makes us want it even more.

My hope is that by this stage of the game your awareness and food sensitivity is heightened to the point where either you will choose not to eat sugar or you will make it the exception rather than the rule. Not because it doesn't taste good, but because it doesn't *feel* good.

The objective, though, is to be able to eat some sugar and get away with it. After all, that's what the corrective counterparts are all about—learning how to make a positive out of a negative.

It sounds awfully complicated. How do I find all these strange fruits?

If you live in a metropolitan area, they should be readily available. Some of the fruits may not be stocked in discount supermarkets, but even then, you may be surprised. To make sure, make your first stop a good market. If you're in a rural area, preorder the fruits through your grocer. They will find them as easy to get as apples and oranges.

Why do you specify dried fruits instead of fresh fruits if we have to put the liquid back in anyway?

You're replacing only part of the moisture, so you're deconcentrating them only slightly—just enough to enable your body to digest them fully. Dried fruits have a much higher concentration of minerals than do fresh fruits, about six times more.

Why can I have butter on my potatoes but not on my popcorn?

I include popcorn in the diet for its ability to act as an intestinal sweep. Butter inhibits this function by slowing down the popcorn's time in your stomach.

Help! I have pimples.

Don't worry. It means you're detoxifying. One of the ways your body eliminates wastes is through your skin. If you break out, it means your skin is eliminating stored toxins, getting rid of the junk inside your body.

All the vitamin A in the mangoes and papaya you're eating will help rectify this. If your skin is breaking out, know that it is only temporary. Once it's over, your complexion will be more glamorous than you ever thought possible. Your new health will manifest itself in your skin. That's one of the marvelous spin-offs of this new way of eating.

Isn't this an expensive way to eat?

No. You might be taken aback by the cost of one papaya, for example, but when you actually figure out what the Beverly Hills Diet costs you each day compared to a day of "traditional" eating, you will find you are spending considerably less.

A staffer of mine who was on the Beverly Hills Diet did a three-month-long cost comparison with her two roommates. The staffer discovered her food costs were 25 percent lower than her roommates'.

When you consider the hidden costs in shopping the old way as well as what you pay for the packaging and preparation of processed foods, it makes sense.

Why would the Beverly Hills Diet work for me when every other diet has been such a failure?

Because this diet is realistic. Unlike other diets, it is not an isolated space in time, a guaranteed number of pounds lost in a specified number of days. It doesn't leave you with a list of maintenance foods that excludes the foods you love.

Instead, you build your world around your favorite foods. What you choose to eat determines what you have to eat. You, in essence, create your own diet. You are not on my diet. You have simply adapted my methodology to *your* diet.

Why don't the other diets work?

Primarily because they include so many nevers. When you go on limited anything, you are bound to lose for a while. The problem is making it last. Portion controls and time limits are self-defeating. When you want a steak, do four ounces really do it for you? Does half a cup of cottage cheese really fill you up? Are you really going to be happy eating carrot sticks and celery indefinitely? Can you honestly agree to never again taste bread and butter, ice cream, cake, or pizza? Other diets create an artificial environment and leave you wanting. They are not and never can be a way of life.

What about orange juice? I thought it was good for you.

There are many fruits that have substantially more vitamin C, such as berries, mangoes, and papaya. Digestively, citrus fruits have few effective enzymes and very little fiber, and they should be eaten only as a last resort and in the morning only. I've experimented extensively with citrus fruits, and the results are conclusive. Not only will you probably not lose, but it is likely that you will gain.

How do I eat when I'm sick?

When we're sick we turn to food from the heart, not from the stomach. Vitamins A and C, which are abundant in fruit, will do far more to nurture you back to health than the nutrients in the traditional "sick" foods like chicken soup or ice cream. Actually, ice cream will aggravate your cold or sore throat by promoting additional mucus secretions. Pineapple, on the other hand, will help dry them up.

If, however, being sick is one of those occasions when you choose to feed your heart rather than your body, go ahead, but *follow the rules.* Remember, sickness is a notorious excuse to blow it, and you no longer need an excuse. Think of it as another opportunity to let your skinny voice prevail.

I'm going into the hospital for an operation. Do I need to take any special dietary precautions?

Most important, *eat exactly as your doctor tells you.* Be aware that there are five times in your life when your need for protein is high—when you're an infant, when you are over sixty-five years of age, when you're pregnant, while you're breast feeding, and before and after surgery.

Because of your increased protein need at this time, I recommend triple protein days (PPP) several days before and several days following your surgery. When ordering from the hospital menu, by all means order low-sodium meals. *But check with your doctor first.*

How fast will I lose weight?

Everyone loses at a different rate, although the average weight loss for the five-week program should balance out.

Clients have lost up to fifteen pounds the first week. The important thing is not how much you lose in a given period of time, but that you *will* lose.

The slowest losers are those whose systems are glutted with salt, chemicals, and sugars. That is the toughest of all combinations for the enzymes to burn through. But ultimately, even these people catch up with the rest.

Can I have fish and meat at the same meal?

Yes. The only protein you can't combine with another protein is nut protein. Combining dairy products with animal proteins should be an exception rather than the rule.

If I don't eat dairy products, where will I get my calcium?

There is calcium in almost everything you eat. You don't really get that much calcium from dairy products anyway, since most of them are indigestible. Those two tablespoons of sesame seeds you now eat each morning have more calcium than two glasses of milk—and they can be fully used by your body because they digest readily.

How much protein should I schedule into a typical week?

At least four to five meals should be protein meals. Don't forget that nuts and avocados are protein foods and a welcome protein change for your body. Keep in mind that protein builds the body. If you are trying to lose weight, do you want to build up your body? Most nutritionists agree that protein plays too great a role in the American diet. Ideally, you should eat about 50 percent carbohydrates, 30 percent fats, and 20 percent protein.

What about mixed nuts?

Acceptable but not advisable. Different tastes, different textures. The tendency will be to overeat. You'll never know when enough is enough.

What about bouillon cubes and consommés?

They are loaded with salt and usually made from beef or chicken stock, so they are not acceptable as a free food or as a base for vegetable soup on a carb night. There is, however, a good low-sodium vegetable bouillon available in health-food stores.

Where does flour fit into the Beverly Hills Diet?

It's a carb and really only combines with other carbs. White flour is the least acceptable because it's nutritionless. Although it's usually enriched, it's still been degrained and debranned. You'll probably find whole-wheat pastry flour to be a happy substitute for baking. Brown-rice flour has a sweet, interesting flavor and is great for breads and tempura. You're much better off buying whole-grain varieties of pasta. It comes in all the same shapes and sizes as the white-flour type.

Forget about soy-flour products. Remember the legume family; they are a miscombination—half protein, half carb—and by their very nature highly indigestible.

My mouth is sore from eating pineapple. What causes it, and what should I do?

It could be caused by any number of things. Usually, it occurs because the pineapple isn't ripe. It will also happen if you eat any of those little eyes or any part of the skin. Even if the skin just touches your mouth, you'll feel it. Try rinsing your mouth out after you eat.

A vitamin B deficiency will also manifest itself as a sore mouth. This will be corrected once nutritional yeast becomes a daily part of your diet.

Do I need to take the supplements even after I've completed Phase Two and am on maintenance?

Yes. You should take them forever. Bran is necessary for its fiber. It's the ultimate nutritional sweep. The yeast keeps your vitamins in balance. And the sesame seeds provide calcium, three essential fatty acids, and more fiber.

Can't J take the yeast in pill form?

No. It doesn't seem to work in any form other than flakes or powder. It is an acquired taste. I've found Kal or Red Star yeast has the best taste. After a while, you'll enjoy it. Try adding only a dash of water so it has a peanut butter consistency and eat it with a spoon. That's how I love it.

What can J drink?

Water, coffee, tea, and uncarbonated water in unlimited amounts. You can also drink wine and fruit and other liquors and beer with carbs as specified by the diet. Nothing alcoholic combines with protein.

Never drink diet soda, which is glutted with chemicals and sodium. Each can has 125 milligrams of sodium—which is about as much as there is in a pound of pork chops!

Js the Beverly Jills Diet okay for children?

Check first, as always, with your doctor. If he/she gives his/her approval and if your child is under fourteen years of age, begin with Week Three.

What if J absolutely have to eat something in the middle of the night?

Eat whatever you last ate before you went to bed. If you're a notorious night eater, it's a good idea to protect yourself by keeping some of the food you last ate in reserve.

When do J begin the "next day"?

Your new day begins when you have gone to sleep for at least five hours. Your pituitary gland, the chief gland in your metabolic process, is most active while you sleep. Most of your hormones are secreted during this period.

I always thought fruit was fattening.

It is if you eat it for dessert. Fruit, remember, can't be digested when eaten after other foods.

What if the Beverly Hills Diet doesn't work for me?

Relax. It will. It works for everyone. All my clients have that fear because it is such a new way of eating.

I hate fruit.

Have you ever eaten a ripe pineapple? Or papaya? Or mango? If all you've ever known in the fruit family are your basic apples and oranges, then you've yet to experience the wonders of this magical kingdom. If you really can't stand the taste of fruit, then obviously this is not the diet for you.

Isn't going without protein unhealthy?

The only kind of protein you are going without is animal protein, and that's only for a brief period. There is some protein in nearly everything you eat. On a watermelon day, for example, you get about twenty-five grams of protein from each watermelon. Incidentally, entire civilizations have existed healthfully without ever eating animal proteins.

What medical reasons would prevent my going on this diet?

If you are hypoglycemic, have ulcers, diabetes, colitis, a spastic colon, or any other serious gastrointestinal problem, or if you are pregnant or breast feeding—then sorry, this diet is not for you. Of course, before beginning any new diet, you should always have a complete physical checkup and get permission from your doctor.

What does pregnancy have to do with anything?

Because this is a cleansing process, toxins will be released into your bloodstream before they're eliminated. You don't want to detoxify or cleanse at this time. Also, don't forget that this is one of the four times in your life when your protein needs, as well as all your other nutritional needs, are unusually high. Don't worry. Papayas will still be here waiting for you when you are ready.

What if I lose too much?

It's essential that you go through the first three weeks of the Beverly Hills Diet and totally detoxify your body. If you should really get too thin, joy of joys you can always gain it back. If at the end of Week One you're at your goal, you could skip Week Two and go on Week Three for two weeks in a row.

When will I know if I've lost enough?

Your best friend, the scale, will tell you. Don't rely on your mirror. And don't succumb to the temptation of listening to your friends. They are used to seeing you fat, and any significant weight loss will impress them. Only you and your scale can make that determination.

When I first decided to go all the way, I thought 105 would be ideal. Once there, I found myself saying, "Well, if I could only lose three more pounds." I had to get to 97 before I was fully convinced I'd arrived. What a thrill being "101 pounds of fun" and a "99-pound weakling!" And what *fun* gaining those five pounds back and settling in at 102. Just as you need to feel what you don't want to be, so you must feel where you do want to be. You must experience that perfect weight.

Do you ever blow it?

Of course, and that's the beauty of my diet. What I've learned to do, however, is use discrimination. I still love pizza, cheesecake, pancakes, spareribs, and french fries. But now I go for the best. If I can't have the best, I simply don't bother. Often, when I give myself permission to blow it, it's unplanned. But it's always with the conviction that I have the corrective counterpart and that I'll use it.

What happens if I don't wait two or three hours before eating different foods?
You'll probably gain weight. It's self-defeating.

Will the Beverly Hills Diet have any effect on my high cholesterol level?
Yes. It will almost inevitably lower it.

In nature, cholesterol appears with lecithin, and the two work together to keep your blood smoothly surging through your body. If the lecithin is missing, cholesterol begins to solidify. Remember, when lecithin is heated it is destroyed. That's why I specify raw nuts, seeds, and butter. That's why I recommend cold-pressed oil. And that's why there's a build-up of cholesterol from roasted nuts and seeds, heat-processed oils, and pasteurized dairy products.

How will it affect high blood pressure?
Because the Beverly Hills Diet excludes salt and chemicals, and because you'll lose weight, your blood pressure should also drop.

What do you eat?
Fruit is still the mainstay of my diet. I begin almost every day with it. But I rarely eat fruit all day. Lunch is often a carb or more fruit and dinner a protein. Dinner typically is an Open Meal, either carb or protein.

I can't believe I won't gain weight if I really eat until I'm full. I'm a big eater.
I honestly doubt you could eat more than I can. Many of my clients initially have this fear, but when you only eat one

thing, it is almost impossible to eat too much of it. One woman ate thirty-six kiwis and eighteen mangoes. She didn't lose, but she didn't gain either. Besides, remember that an important process of the Beverly Hills Diet is *feeding* your body, not starving it.

I'm taking medication. Should I stop? Will it interfere with my weight loss?

It's hard to say whether it will interfere. But do not stop taking any medication your doctor has prescribed for you. Always follow your doctor's instructions.

A last-minute invitation came up, and it's my favorite restaurant. I'm on a grape day. Now what?

Stay on your grapes and know the restaurant will still be there tomorrow. It's only your favorite because you have been there before and you'll go there again. Remember, if you give in to every last-minute invitation, there's only one thing that will disappear, and that's your newfound hipbones.

What should I do about my headache?

First, try eating. Headaches are often a sign of hunger. If the headache appears for the first few days of the Beverly Hills Diet, it may be a sign that your body is detoxifying. It will go away. If you absolutely must take an aspirin then go ahead, but try not to. You'll survive.

Can I use a breath spray?

Unfortunately, all breath sprays, mints, and washes are swarming with chemicals, sugar, and sodium. Eating the way you do as a Conscious Combiner, you have no need for breath camouflages anyway.

What about diuretics?

If they have been prescribed for you by your doctor, continue taking them. If, on the other hand, you are taking them as a diet ploy, stop. This diet has natural diuretics built in at the appropriate stages of your weight-loss schedule. The pills rob your body of vital nutrients. If you are giving up diuretics, hooray, but be prepared for a slightly slower start in your weight loss as your body adjusts. Don't let it throw you. You'll catch up, I promise.

Are there any limits on the amount of oil I can use?

No. Remember that oil is a fat and thus digests with anything. It also provides your body with the three fatty acids you can only obtain from food.

When you heat oil, don't you destroy its key digestive enzyme, lecithin?

Yes. Use as little as possible for cooking. If you are adding oil for flavor, add it after the food is cooked. By the way, oil should never be reused because each time it is reheated more and more of its life-giving properties are destroyed.

Won't I lose more weight if I continue to just eat fruit?

No. Man does not live by pineapple alone. Once your body is cleansed, it is the proper balance of all different types of foods, the combination of nutrients from many different sources that will allow you to achieve maximum weight loss. Don't perpetuate your former imbalance by creating a new one.

What are the biggest problems your clients have?

Not eating enough the first week. It's hard letting go of the old diet consciousness that dieting is synonomous with deprivation and hunger. They don't yet understand that the burn, feed, and wash process depends on feeding their bodies. It takes a while to accept the power of those enzymes. They also have a hard time giving up total control of the most important thing in their life—food. The third biggest problem is internalizing the fact that this is a way of eating forever, experiencing the concept of tomorrow.

If something comes up at the last minute, can I switch the order of the Beverly Hills Diet days to accommodate my new plans?

Not on the Five-Week Beverly Hills Diet. Often it's the combination of two days of foods that makes the third day work. Foods are given in a specific order for specific reasons. Don't upset the enzyme balance. It's only one day in a lifetime.

What about all the people who miscombine like crazy and never get fat?

Watch them carefully. They are different. I would guess there are often times when they simply forget to eat. Something we eaters never do. And when they do eat, they do so with moderation, knowing when enough is enough. Something we eaters don't know.

For one reason or another their bodies somehow don't process their food into fat. But then again they don't love food the way we do. When food is in their mouths their hearts don't sing and their souls don't soar. They aren't so lucky; look at the enjoyment they are missing out on. I would guess that most of those people do have indigestion from their miscombining. It just manifests itself in ways other than fat.

XII

Welcome to the World of the Little Golden Pineapple

Tomorrow is here. Here for you to celebrate. Could you have imagined getting on your scale and not having to lose one more pound? Could you have imagined being perfect? Did you ever realize how much of your life was colored by fat?

Did you ever imagine a tomorrow that includes everything you ever wanted to eat? Being able to eat to your heart's content—without eating your heart out? Did you ever imagine a tomorrow when you would be totally in control, when the old diet consciousness would be banished forever? Did you ever think you'd be able to make food work for *you*—not by giving it up but just by unlocking its enzymes?

At long last, you can have your cake and eat it too. Does it really matter if you have to eat it one piece at a time? One by one, all your excuses have been stripped away. There's nothing out there you can't eat. Nothing. You've eliminated your greatest obstacle to slimhood: you.

Gone forever is the fat consciousness, the wallowing in self-pity, the obsession with negatives. Gone forever is the desperation, the desolation, the resignation, and the guilt of being fat forever. No longer does skinny mean hunger, deprivation, and a black cloud of nevers. No longer will food sap your power and energy. You have learned how to manipulate food, how to use it to maximize your energy, how to use food to keep you thin.

Here forever is a reality that includes everything you ever wanted. A diet that is, in fact, a way of life, a dream come true. A diet where nothing is fattening, a diet that builds in antidotes for blowing it, in which, no matter what you eat, there's a corrective counterpart to erase its effects. A diet that feeds your body instead of starving it.

For the first time in your life you have permission to enjoy food, to make food an experience and to experience food. For the first time in your life, you have embraced a way of eating that is built around the foods you love. What you choose to eat determines what you have to eat. You never have to cheat to get what you want, because there's no diet to break. This is *your* diet, not somebody else's. And it's forever.

You don't have to prove anything anymore. You have made a commitment that means always. You have put your mind and your intellect into eating. You have learned to make conscious choices. You have shed the fat-perpetuating diet consciousness forever.

For the first time in your life you have glorious energy, a body you can be proud of, and the ammunition to keep it that way for the rest of your life.

Two of my famous clients put it in their own words. From John Wayne's granddaughter, Teresa Wayne: "The marvelous thing about Judy's plan of eating is that I never felt like I was on a *diet*. I never felt deprived, like I did on all my other diets. I knew if I wanted something . . . I could have it. I learned to taste new foods and eat in a whole different way. I'm thin now and am keeping my weight down on my own. I'm happy being skinny, and I won't ever be fat again, thanks to Judy!"

Says Engelbert Humperdinck, "For years I've been guilty of being undisciplined in eating and drinking anything and everything. Until one day I looked in the mirror and realized with disgust that I'd thrown my self-pride out of the window. Following a visit to my dentist, who informed me he had lost 13½ pounds in one week, I asked for the remedy. He replied with a name—Judy Mazel. I immediately visited this lady and found her to be just that. A lady of concern, and to coin a phrase, she puts her money where her mouth is. In 4½ weeks I lost 31 pounds. No drugs, by that I mean no diet pills, etc. . . . , no starvation—just a healthy program of nutritious foods. I went from a 36-inch waist to a 29. My tailor was unhappy, but I was delighted. Now when I look in the mirror I feel proud to have had the opportunity to meet a lady, and her diet, called Judy Mazel. My sincere thanks."

One American in five is fat. Are you one of them? If you're not skinny, if you're not yet perfect, make a commitment to me for five weeks. I'm not going to take your food away from you. I'm not going to make you give up eating. I'm not going to make you say goodbye to your hamburger with everything on it, your pizza, or your apple pie. I'm going to show you how to enjoy them, enjoy food—all food—without guilt. I am going to teach you how to get away with murder and not serve a life sentence. This is it, the end of the line. Relax, experience, and enjoy.

Since you can't imagine living without the foods you love, isn't it about time you created your world around those foods? Follow my path to discovery, and create a new diet reality, a skinny reality. The time is now.

If you have any questions about the Beverly Hills Diet, if you have any problems, if you feel the diet is not working for you, go back and reread this book carefully. This is a new way of eating based on the physical laws that govern your body. For it to succeed, you must understand how and why it works, and you must follow the commandments and rules exactly as they are outlined. Any variance can offset the balances and cause the diet to fail.

If you still have questions, I encourage you to write me.

I'd like to extend a special invitation to those of you who successfully complete the first two phases of the Beverly Hills Diet and maintain your weight loss for thirty days.

Keep a record of your weight loss through the five-week program until you reach your goal weight and then through the first month of maintenance. Record not only your weight, but what you eat each day once you are on maintenance.

Send me a copy of these records, and I will welcome you into the family of Beverly Hills Conscious Combiners with a little golden pineapple, our symbol of eternal slimhood. More important, when you send me your records, you will be linking up with our nationwide network of Conscious Combiners. You will become an important part of a support system that will help keep you skinny forever.

The Beverly Hills Diet is indeed the way of life for the '80s. Tomorrow is here, and it is here for you to enjoy. Join us in the world of the little skinny pineapple.

Write:

Judy Mazel
The Beverly Hills Diet
270 N. Cañon Dr.
Beverly Hills, California 90210

Glossary

AMINO ACIDS Building blocks derived from protein sources

ANIMAL PROTEIN Protein derived from animal sources

BALANCED DIET A regimen in which you are getting the proper balance of nutrients to promote and maintain health and slimness

BEVERLY HILLS DIET PROCESS, THE Includes burn, feed, and wash

- *Burning* is the process in which enzymes are used to burn up and digest fat and extra protein.

- *Feeding* is the process in which minerals are being supplied to your body in highly concentrated doses to offset a mineral imbalance and to reestablish the harmony of the cells.

- *Washing* is the process in which fruit is used to eliminate extra fluid, chemicals, burned-up fat, and protein from your body.

BLOWING IT Miscombining either with or without permission

BRAN Flakes derived from wheat or rice. The outer fibrous hull is used by the body as an elimination aid.

BROMALINE The active enzyme in pineapple and strawberries, which interacts with and stimulates the hydrochloric acid in the stomach to digest fat

CARBOHYDRATES Carbohydrates break down into glucose, which provides our body with energy. They are our fuel, the gasoline on which we run.

CLEANSING Detoxifying. The process whereby toxins are eliminated by

249

our bodies. It's accomplished on the Beverly Hills Diet through the burn, feed, and wash process.

COLD-PRESSED OIL Sometimes called expellor pressed. Processed oil extracted from its source by a pressing method rather than a heating method.

CONSCIOUS COMBINER Person who combines food to achieve the ultimate nutritional value afforded by those foods. A person who knows what digests well together and what doesn't and who chooses to eat accordingly.

CORRECTIVE COUNTERPARTS Digestive foods that interact and offset previously eaten hard-to-digest foods.

DAIRY PROTEINS Proteins derived from dairy sources, such as milk, cheese, eggs, and yogurt.

DIGESTIVE PROCESS The process whereby your body uses and processes food to maintain life and to provide it with energy

- *Digestion.* Step one in the digestive process. The stage at which food is turned into nutrients.
- *Absorption.* Step two in the digestive process. The stage at which all nutrients are absorbed into the blood and sent to the cells.
- *Metabolism.* Step three in the digestive process. The stage at which all our cells are nourished and our body burns up energy.
- *Elimination.* Step four in the digestive process. The stage at which the unused waste products are eliminated. The main vehicles of elimination are urination, bowel movements, perspiration, and breathing.

DISTILLED SPIRITS Includes all grain alcohols—vodka, tequila, bourbon, scotch, rye, sake, and beer

ENZYMATICALLY OPEN A condition in which you have not limited yourself to having to eat a specific food

ENZYMES Little chemical reactors that speed up chemical reactions in our bodies. They either appear in the food we eat or are promoted in our bodies by the food we eat. Enzymes take human food and turn it into body food.

FAT   When you have five pounds or fifty pounds to lose. Fat is whenever you can't get on the scale and say "I'm perfect."

FAT CONSCIOUSNESS   That self-perpetuating way of thinking that makes us and keeps us fat

FATS   Fats ultimately break down into lipids, the carriers of vitamins A, D, E, and K. They provide our body with stored energy.

FATTENING   Foods that are hard to digest or indigestible

GLUCOSE   The energy form derived from carbohydrates

HERB   A plant valued for its flavor and scent; used for seasoning or medicinal properties. Examples: basil, oregano, rosemary, and thyme.

HYDROCHLORIC ACID   The digestive enzyme that digests fat in our stomach

INDIGESTIBLE   Those foods that are impossible for our body to break down into nutrients because of the combination in which they are ingested or because of their intrinsic molecular makeup. These foods ultimately become clogged in our bodies and cause our fat.

LAST SUPPER   Eating as if it's the last meal of your life

LECITHIN_   An essential fatty acid, a natural substance that always appears in conjunction with cholesterol. It's not only found in food, but is present in every cell in your body, particularly in your nervous system. Its action is that of an emulsifier. It is the essential part of fat that allows it to be digested.

LEGUMES   A food category made up of foods that are half protein and half carbohydrate. They are highly indigestible because of their innate miscombination.

LIPIDS   Stored energy derived from fat sources

MAINTENANCE   That forever period of perfection when eternal slimhood is a reality

MALTOSE   A sugar formed by the first stage of carbohydrate digestion

MARTYR   A person who sits at the table and just drinks coffee or tea while watching everyone else eat and saying he isn't hungry when he is

MAXI CARBS   Molecularly speaking, the most complex category of carbs. Also known as the starches because of their complexity and because they can be converted into flour. They take the longest of all the carbs to digest.

MENSCH   A human being

MIDI CARBS   Carbs with a molecular structure more complex than that of the simpler mini carbs but not as complex as the maxi carbs

MIND/BODY SPLIT   When the mind and the body are disconnected; a condition in which you don't feel your body or experience it as it really is

MINERALS   Inorganic compounds necessary for life

MINI CARBS   The most easily digested of all the carbohydrates

MISCOMBINATION   Combining proteins and carbohydrates at the same time

MISHAMISHIMA   A total miscombination—sugar, salt, chemicals, grease, the works. Its literal translation: a strange death.

MONO MEAL   A meal consisting of a single food

NUT PROTEIN   Protein derived from nuts and seeds, including avocados

NUTRIENTS   Vitamins, minerals, amino acids, glucose, and lipids. Nutrients are body food.

NUTRITIONAL YEAST   An inactive yeast specifically designed as a food supplement to provide the body with B vitamins, amino acids, and minerals

OPEN CARB   A combination of three carbs, not more than two of which are maxi carbs

OPEN DESSERT   Dessert instead of a meal. If it is in lieu of a midday meal, two human portions of any dessert you choose. If it is in lieu of an evening meal, three human portions of any dessert.

OPEN FRUIT   Fruit combined with wine, champagne, or brandy. One fruit only. Fruits do not combine with one another.

OPEN HUMAN   Eating like a mensch (see "MENSCH" above) with one hand and one bite at a time while watching a skinny person and imitating him or her bite for bite

OPEN MEAL—Meals not restricted to a single food

OPEN MISCOMBINATION   There are two types:

1. One protein and one carb. Follow the rule of eating the protein

last. Eat the carb first, and once you've taken your first bite of protein, don't go back to the carb.

2. Those foods—entities unto themselves—that contain both a protein and a carb and thus exist only as a miscombination. (*see* MISCOMBINATION above)

OPEN PROTEIN   The combination of any three proteins from any category, excluding nuts. Nut proteins combine with nothing.

ORGANIC   Natural, without chemicals or preservatives

PAPAIN   The active enzyme in papaya, mango, kiwi, and persimmon. It interacts with and promotes the secretion of pepsin in our stomach to digest protein.

PRECIDOTE   Opposite of an antidote; it preceeds, or comes before a meal and enzymatically prepares you for it.

PROTEIN   Proteins break down into amino acids, the building blocks from which our flesh, blood, and muscles are made.

PTYALIN   The enzyme secreted in the saliva and promoted by chewing that is essential for the digestion of carbohydrates

RAW BUTTER   Butter made from unpasteurized milk

RESNICK OPEN   Drinking instead of eating

SESAME SEEDS   A high-protein, high-calcium, high-fiber food which is an important part of the Beverly Hills Diet

SKINNY VOICE   When your head says no and your heart says go, it's the voice that stops you

SUCROSE   The sugar obtained from sugarcane or sugar beets

SWEETENERS   All sugars, syrups, and honey

TOXINS   Poisons, the residue of which is trapped in our bodies because of uneliminated waste products and chemicals

"TRADITIONAL" BALANCED DIET   Breakfast, lunch, and dinner or eating proteins, carbs, and fats at the same meal

VICTIM   One who unnecessarily places himself in a potentially fattening position

VITAMINS   Compounds necessary for the maintenance of life

WHOLE GRAINS   Unrefined grains from which the germ and the bran have not been removed

Index

Beverly Hills Diet (*continued*)
  maintenance program in, *see*
    maintenance program
  in middle of the night, 238
  moderation and, 92–93, 103–104,
    109, 113, 129
  never-permitted foods in, 37–38
  "next day" defined in, 238–239
  nonphysical exercises in, 60, 69,
    70, 77, 84, 99, 104, 107,
    127–128
  phase one of, 58–85
  phase two of, 86–108
  phase three of, 109–115
  physical exercise and, 126–127
  pitfalls to avoid in, 132–141, 235
  plateaus as peril in, 132–137
  questions often asked about,
    229–244
  rate of loss expected in, 235–236
  as realistic, 234
  recipes for, 174–202
  restaurants and, 213–225
  rules for phase one, 60–62
  rule stretching in, 90, 130–131,
    145–150, 154, 157
  serving styles and, 171–173
  for social occasions, 203–212
  substitute list for phase one,
    62–63
  supplements in phase two, 87
  temporary physical discomforts in,
    123–124, 231, 233, 242
  Ten Commandments in, 56–57
  time off from, 108, 109, 113, 137,
    240–241
  too great weight loss in, 240
  in traveling, 224–228
  tricks and tips for, 124–141
  waiting time between changes of
    food in, 61, 66, 75, 241, 244
  when inappropriate, 60, 239
  when-to-eat principle in, 21
  when to repeat specific weeks of
    diet, 115

birthdays, to celebrate "born-again
  skinny," 211
Bjorg Special, 218
Blount, Bill, 138
Blowing It Without Blowing It, 109,
  137, 140, 240–241
Blumberg, Philip, 225
body processes, four stages of, 22,
  23–25
Bogart, Neil, 138, 173
bouillon cubes, 237
bran, 46, 87, 237
brandy, 89, 157
bread, white, 46, 237
breakfast:
  choice of fruit for, 226
  traditional, 105
breath sprays, 242
bromaline (enzyme), 67
Brown, Sam, 216
butter:
  raw, unsalted, 171
  when to use, 233
B vitamins:
  sugar and, 45
  supplements of, 48, 87, 237–238

calcium, 40–41, 87, 236
Calendo, John, 2–3
calories, 28
  in "low-cal" diets, 49
  percentages in balanced diet of,
    31
carbohydrates:
  in combined meals, 89, 93
  complex, digestion of, 35
  correction food-group combina-
    tions for, 36–37
  in digestive process, 23, 35, 156–
    157, 237
  enzymes related to, 22, 23, 33–34,
    35
  foods classified as, 31
  glucose and, 28
  in maintenance program, 150–153
  mini, midi, and maxi, 32

protein and, 34, 36–37
refined, 44–46
sweeteners and, 34
see also combined meals
carbonated beverages, 157
case histories, 2–3, 8–9
of Hollywood stars, 5–7
of Judy Mazel, 10–20
champagne, 89, 157
cheating, 140–141, 227, 231
see also guilt; nibbling; perfectionism
cheese, 40–41, 156, 218
chewing, of carbohydrates, 33–34, 172
chicken, 51, 82–83
children, Beverly Hills Diet and, 238
Chinese restaurants, pros and cons of, 220–221
Chinese restaurant syndrome, 220
chips, unsalted, 171
cholesterol, 47, 241
citrus fruit, 50, 67, 226
coffee, 158, 238
combined meals, 86, 88–93
correctives for, 37, 90–91, 93, 97, 126, 130, 140, 146–150, 156, 231, 232
drinking and, 89, 91, 97, 157, 205, 238
Open Carb, 89, 93, 98, 150, 151
Open Dessert in, 91, 151
Open Fruit, 89, 97, 150, 151
Open Human in, 91–93, 129, 151
Open Miscombination in, 90–91, 93, 97, 151
Open Protein, 89, 90–91, 93, 150, 151
Resnick Open in, 91, 97, 151, 205–206
special recoups and, 149
see also miscombinations
Conscious Combining Technique:
basic principles of, 18–20, 36–37
functioning of, see Beverly Hills Diet

see also combined meals
consommés, 237
corn, as intestinal sweep, 76
corrective counterparts, 37, 90–91, 93, 97, 126, 130, 140, 146–150, 156, 231, 232
cottage cheese, as "diet," 49
cruises, cheating and, 227

dairy products, 41–42, 46, 49, 158, 171, 236
in digestive process, 35, 39, 40
as protein, 31
diarrhea, 231
diet foods, as fattening, 49
diet pills, 11, 12
diets, other:
as myths, 48–52
reasons for failure of, 234
diet soda, 37–38, 64, 157, 238
digestion:
basic laws of, 15
as stage of digestive process, 23–24
weight control and, 16
see also undigested food
digestive process and system, 15, 21–26
diuretics, 12, 242–243

eggs, 50–51
elimination, 124, 231
in digestive process, 25
fiber and, 25, 46, 50, 51, 87, 172, 237–238
foods hindering, 41, 45
through skin, 233
water and, 43
emotional eaters, 16–17, 19, 52–57, 130
feeling and, 54–55, 122–124, 128, 137–141, 142–144, 243–244
personality of, 52–53, 145
energy, 36, 122–124, 230
from carbohydrates vs. proteins, 28, 155

energy (*continued*)
  diet foods and, 50, 51
  emotional eating and, 54
  equating food with, 57, 122
enzymes, 230
  as antagonists, 22, 33–35
  clocking action of, 35–37
  in maintenance program, 146–147,
    154
  pivotal role of, 15, 17, 19, 22, 231
  specific functions of, 22
  in tropical fruits, 18, 58, 63, 67

fat, body:
  undigested food as cause of, 21,
    25–26, 36
  water in, 43
fatigue, *see* energy
fat people:
  confronting and letting go of
    weight by, 57, 59, 60, 99, 128,
    131, 135
  excuses by, 137–139
  fighting failure consciousness by,
    69, 84, 139–140
  rejecting skinny selves by,
    139–140
fats, dietary:
  correct food-group combinations
    for, 36–37
  in digestive process, 23, 35–36
  enzymes related to, 22, 23
  foods classified as, 31
fatty acids, 87, 238, 243
fiber, 25, 46, 50, 51, 87, 172, 237–
  238
Fields, Totie, 136
figs, 168
flour, 237
food-awareness training, 53–55, 59,
  122, 232
food groups, classification of, 30–31
French restaurants, pros and cons
  of, 216, 217–218
fruit:
  canned, 169–170

in carbohydrate classification, 31
citrus, 50, 67, 226, 234–235
in combined meals, 89
in digestive process, 23–24, 36
dried, 73–74, 154–155, 169, 170,
  233
enzymatic, 18, 58, 63, 66–67
frozen, 169, 170
fruit haters and, 239
illness and, 235
as juice, 172, 234–235
in maintenance program, 150–153,
  154
minerals in, 73, 233
neutral, 19, 155, 226
non-combination principle for, 36,
  89
in phase one, 58–59
in phase two, 86
ripeness of, 165, 168–169
serving styles for, 171–173
shopping for, 165–170, 232–233
to start 80% of days' eating, 226
when fattening, 239
see also specific fruits

gas, intestinal, 25, 124, 155
Gershen, Scott, 14
glucose, 22, 27–28, 45, 231–232
Gold, Jerry, 140
golden pineapple award, 248
Goldstein, Patrick, 5
grapefruit, 50, 226
grapes, 74, 156, 168
  as all-day fruits, 154, 226
Gray, Linda, 6, 156
guilt, fat consciousness and, 92,
  139–140

habits, bad, overcoming of, 136–137
hamburger, as "diet," 49
Harrington, Pat, 5–6, 156
Haymer, Susan, 5, 215–216
headaches, 242
high blood pressure, 43, 241

holidays:
    eating choices on, 208–212
    recoups for, 149
Humperdinck, Englebert, 127, 227,
    246–247
hydrochloric acid (enzyme func-
    tioning), 22, 23, 34, 67

illnesses, 235
indigestion, causes of, 25, 36, 244
Italian restaurants, pros and cons
    of, 218–219

Japanese restaurants, pros and cons
    of, 221
jet lag, 225
jobs, bringing fruit to, 173
juices, fruit, 172, 234–235

Kellerman, Sally, 4, 6, 227
kiwis, 67, 167

"last supper" attitude, 19, 109, 141
lecithin, 39, 41, 46, 47, 50, 241, 243
legumes, 30, 33, 237
lemons, 50, 67, 230
limes, 50, 67, 230
lipids, 22, 23, 28
liquors, what to eat with, 91, 157,
    205–206, 238

maintenance program, 85, 115,
    142–163
    appropriate correctives in, see
        corrective counterparts
    daily combinations for, 150–154
    dangerous foods and combos in,
        157–159
    experimenting and, 145–150, 154,
        157
    fixed rules in, 154
    general rules in, 154–157
    special recoups in, 149
    three-part-day plan in, 148–149,
        152–153
    weekly charting of, 159–163

maltose, 23, 33
mangoes, 18, 67, 233
    shopping for, 166
Martin, Dick, 204
maxi carbs, 32, 155
medication, dieting and, 242–243
melons, 51, 226
metabolism, in digestive process, 24
Mexican restaurants, pros and cons
    of, 221–222
midi carbs, 32
milk, 39–40, 46, 158
mind/body split, 14, 52–55, 127–
    128, 129, 134–135, 137–140, 228
minerals, 22, 24, 26–27, 40–41, 87,
    236
    in fruits, 73, 233
mineral water, 44, 157, 238
mini carbs, 32
mirrors, full-length, 84
miscombinations:
    correcting of, 37, 90–91, 93, 97,
        126, 130, 140, 146–150, 156,
        231, 232
    foods causing, 37–46
    precidotes for, 155, 206
    special meals as, 149, 208–212
    thin people's response to, 244
mishamishima, 149
Mobley, Mary Ann, 7
Molasky, Irwin, 138
Mono Meals, 88, 93, 151, 152, 216
    for weight loss, 93, 217
Mono Protein Meal, 91, 93, 105–106
mouth:
    in digestive process, 23
    soreness of, from pineapple, 237
MSG (monosodium glutamate), 220,
    221
Muldaur, Maria, 4

nibbling, 136, 206, 231
nutrients, 21–22
    in digestive process, 21–26
    function of, 26–30